Women in Later Life

Exploring 'Race' and Ethnicity

D0145373

Women in Later Life

Exploring 'Race' and Ethnicity

by
Mary Maynard, Haleh Afshar,
Myfanwy Franks and Sharon Wray

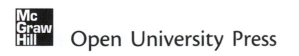
McGraw Hill

Open University Press

Open University Press
McGraw-Hill Education
McGraw-Hill House
Shoppenhangers Road
Maidenhead
Berkshire
England
SL6 2QL
email: enquiries@openup.co.uk
world wide web: www.openup.co.uk

and Two Penn Plaza, New York, NY 10121-2289, USA

First published 2008

Copyright ©

All rights reserved. Except for the quotation of short passages for the purposes of
criticism and review, no part of this publication may be reproduced, stored in a retrieval
system, or transmitted, in any form, or by any means, electronic, mechanical,
photocopying, recording or otherwise, without the prior permission of the publisher or
a licence from the Copyright Licensing Agency Limited. Details of such licences (for
reprographic reproduction) may be obtained from the Copyright Licensing Agency Ltd
of 90 Tottenham Court Road, London, W1T 4LP.

A catalogue record of this book is available from the British Library

ISBN-10: 0-335-21525-4 (pb), 0-355-21526-2 (hb)
ISBN-13: 978-0-335-21525-6 (pb), 978-0-335-21526-3 (hb)

Library of Congress Cataloging-in-Publication Data
CIP data applied for

Typeset by YHT Ltd, London
Printed in Great Britain by Bell and Bain Ltd., in Glasgow

The *McGraw·Hill* Companies

Contents

Handwritten annotations: Module 2 (next to 2), Module 1 (next to 3), Module 4 to 5 (next to 5), Module 3 (next to 8)

Acknowledgements

Our thanks go to all the women who gave up their time to tell us their stories, aspects of which for some were harrowing to relive.

We are also grateful to community leaders and members who helped us gain access to our participants and to those who acted as interpreters.

The research was funded by a grant from the Economic and Social Research Council number L 480 25 4047.

1

Introduction

The UK, along with other Western and industrialized countries, has an aging population. We already live in one of the oldest societies to have ever existed and it is going to get older. The 2001 Census shows that for the first time there are more people over 60 years of age (21 percent of the population) than under 16 (20 percent) (ONS 2003). By 2020 it is estimated that one-third of the population will be aged over 50. Yet, while it might be thought that the fact that people are living longer would be cause for celebration, there has been a tendency instead for an ethos of gloom and doom to exist. As the Director of the Economic and Social Research Council's (ESRC) research series, the Growing Older Programme, has put it, the debate is frequently filled, 'by a demography of despair, which portrays population aging not as a triumph for civilization, but as something closer to an apocalypse' (Walker 2001).

The research upon which this book is based was conducted as part of the Growing Older Programme. The latter consisted of 24 projects spread across six topics deemed to be central to extending quality of life: defining and measuring it; inequalities in quality of life; technology and the built environment; healthy and productive aging; family and support networks; and participation and activity in later life. Our research was located in the latter stream although, as with all the projects, its focus necessarily strayed into the others.

This introduction aims to do three things. First, it looks in more detail at what is involved in the aging process that is taking place. It then provides some information about the nature of our research, why it was undertaken and what was actually done. Finally, it gives an overview of research findings and explains the structure of the book and the content of the chapters that follow.

An aging population

As explained above, one of the greatest achievements of the last century must be the 25 years that have been added to life expectancy (Dean n.d.). Further, the population has grown by 6.5 percent in the last thirty or so years, from 55.9 million in 1971 to 59.6 million by mid-2003 (ONS 2003). However, as has already been intimated, the increases that have taken place have not occurred at all ages. While the proportion of those aged 65 and over has increased, the numbers of those aged 16 and younger has decreased and is less now than it was 30 years ago. The proportion of those in the 65 plus age bracket increased from 13 percent in mid-1971 to 16 percent in mid-2003. During the same period, there was a fall in the percentage of those aged 16 years or under from 25 to 20 percent (ONS 2003).

One of the reasons why these demographic changes have not been greeted with unbounded enthusiasm is due to the implications they are said to have for the dependency ratio (Phillipson 1998; Street and Ginn, 2001). The latter measures the proportion of those who are dependant in a population (children and pensioners) in relation to the number of those of working age. The problem is seen to be that this ratio is increasing and is projected to continue to do so. This means that there are fewer people who are economically active and yet it is this activity, through the payment of taxes and so on, which supports those who are 'dependant', in the case of older people through the provision of pensions and other kinds of social support. This raises questions about the extent to which the welfare state can continue to make provision at current levels. What has been termed 'the generational contract', whereby the state provides security in later life in return for services (for instance in times of war) and economic contributions made while working, is seen to be in jeopardy. While many later life researchers have been questioning the extent to which this is actually the case, a 'demographic time bomb', leading to a crisis in the welfare state, is often how the issue of aging is addressed, by both politicians and the media (Walker 1996; Phillipson 1998; Arber and Attias-Donfut 2000).

Yet, as some have pointed out, discussion often overlooks issues such as the (potential) increased productivity of those who work, together with the fact that retirement is no longer defined only by age and a range of pathways out of the workplace have emerged (Phillipson 1998, 2004). It is also the case that there are political choices to be made between raising taxes and national insurance contributions and/ or the retirement age or reducing welfare state provision and encouraging individuals to fund services privately. All these courses of action are, of course, hotly debated. What is not often discussed, however, is how such debates tend to exclude the position of women (Arber and Attias-Donfut 2000). This is because, as Street and Ginn put it, 'women "disappear" when populations are considered in the aggregate, yet are intrinsically linked to population aging' (2001: 35). The current generation of elderly women were present at the establishment of the welfare state, when notions about retirement and pensions were 'developed by men with men in mind' (Hill and Tigges, 1995: 100). Due to part-time working, lower wages and reduced rate contributions for those who were married, women may find themselves seriously financially disadvantaged in their later years. This particularly becomes an issue, given the numbers of elderly women who are present in the UK today and their greater likelihood of living in poverty (see Chapter 2).

According to ONS statistics, there were 12.5 million men aged between 60 and 74 years in 2001 and 3 012 100 aged 75 and over (ONS 2003). This contrasts with the numbers for women, which were 16.6 million and 5 606 600 respectively. It can, therefore, be seen that there are over a quarter more elderly women than men in the former age group and getting on for nearly twice as many in the latter. When it comes to those who are aged over 90, the numbers for men and for women are, again, 100 400 and 317 800 respectively, more than three times as many. These figures have implications for gender inequalities and for the quality of life of older women, which is discussed in the next chapter. Older women out number older men, since men tend to die at a younger age than women. The fact that the number of women compared to men is so pronounced among the very old is because the former tend to live longer than the latter. ONS expectation of life tables indicate that while at 60 a woman could expect to live for another 23.6 years, the expectation of life for a man of the same age is 20 years (Age Concern 2007). The death of men in the First and Second World Wars has also had an impact on this demographic profile. In recent years an improvement in the death rate for older men has led to a narrowing of the gender gap between older men and women. Although projections suggest a further narrowing of this gap by 2031, it will still remain a significant gender difference in terms of later life (ONS 2003).

Of course, the above figures represent the situation taken for the population as a whole and they need to be disaggregated further if important aspects of difference and diversity are to be taken into account. The 2001 Census indicates that the category 'white' accounted for 92.1 percent of the population size in the UK, with minority ethnic groups comprising 4.6 million or 7.9 percent of the total (ONS 2003). Indians formed the largest category, followed by Pakistanis, those of mixed ethnic backgrounds, black Caribbeans, black Africans and Bangladeshis. It is also the case that minority ethnic groups tend to have a younger age structure than the white population, although their progressive aging is anticipated. This reflects past immigration and fertility patterns. The first large-scale migration of people of ethnic minority origin came from the West Indian islands shortly after the Second World War and during the 1950s. Polish migrants also arrived during this period. Immigrants came from India and Pakistan mainly during the 1960s. Most of those with a Bangladeshi background arrived during the 1970s (Bloch 2002).The black Caribbean population is the most elderly minority ethnic group, with 11 percent aged over 65 and will contain substantial numbers of elderly people from 2010 onwards. For other groups the figures for those over 65 are Indians 7 percent, Chinese 5 percent, Pakistani 4 percent, Bangladeshi 3 percent, and Black African people 2 percent (National Statistics 2006). However, it has been estimated that there are now over 350 000 people aged 65 and over from minority ethnic communities and that this is more than twice the number who existed in 1991 (White 2002).

For minority ethnic groups, as with the white population, differences in mortality rates usually mean that women aged 65 and over out-number men. However, for some ethnic groups, this has been influenced by different and gendered migration patterns. This is particularly the case for Bangladeshi older people, where the Census indicates that only one-third (34 percent) of those aged 65 plus were women (ONS 2003). Similarly, in the Pakistani group women comprised 45 percent of those within this age category. Thus, the demographic profile of older people in general, in the UK, and older women in particular is complex. They are not a homogeneous group.

However, this heterogeneity often goes unrecognized in studies of later life. This then provided the starting point for our research.

A qualitative study of gender, ethnic differences and later life

Our research with older women had two main points of departure. The first was our agreement with those who have been critical of the overly problematizing and welfarist approach that has tended to be used in the study of aging (Phillipson 1998; Maynard 1999). While there is a research obligation not to minimize the real social and economic difficulties that face significant numbers of older people, there is also a need to explore the more positive aspects of later life and how these might be facilitated and supported. Rather than treating older people and older women in particular, as the sources of social policy problems, we need also to investigate the circumstances that enhance their ability to pursue their lives.

The second impetus was a desire to contribute to the growing body of knowledge on older women's experiences in later life. Since the publication of Arber and Ginn's path-breaking, *Gender and Later Life*, in 1991, many other studies about the gendered nature of the aging process have been undertaken, with an expansion of interest and writing on the topic. However, this is still not necessarily seen as a mainstream part of social gerontology. Further, in some quarters there has been a tendency to treat gender simply as a variable, rather than as a social attribute that qualitatively affects the experience of aging. In addition, despite being resident in the UK for anything up to 50 years and the fact that they too are aging, relatively little is known about the elderly from the minority ethnic communities. Much of the research that exists has been funded on a shoestring by service providers and has largely been directed at discovering participants' knowledge about specific forms of local provision (Butt and Moriarty 2005). In the past, there also seems to have been an assumption that minority ethnic groups have their needs catered for by their extended family and kin network (Katbamna 2004).

For these reasons we undertook qualitative interviews and focus groups with older women from the African-Caribbean, Asian, Polish and white non-migrant communities. The two central questions were:

how do older women understand and evaluate their quality of life and how might this quality be extended? The term 'quality of life' has entered everyday usage and there is disagreement as to what it means and how it might be measured (Smith 2000a, b, 2001; Butt and Moriarty 2005). Here we concentrated on how our contributors understood the term themselves and the things that they attributed to it. It was our original intention to recruit women between the ages of 60 and 75. Most of our contributors do fall into this age group. However, there are also two who are 58 and some in their later 70s and even in their 80s. This was because it proved difficult to turn away women, who clearly saw their lives as relevant to the study, when they appeared for focus groups and interviews. Indeed, some of the respondents from the Indian subcontinent had no birth certificates and were not entirely sure how old they were.

The research was located in the north of England and participants were recruited via community leaders, centres and groups. In one sense this was not ideal. Others have pointed to the dangers that lie within such a strategy. This includes discouraging participation for fear that such gatekeepers may find out about and then divulge what has been said (Letherby 2003). There is also the likely possibility that the gate-keepers themselves might try to influence the research, particularly in relation to how they select participants or draw up a list of names from which the researchers are to select (Reynolds 2002). However, since only one of the four researchers in our team was from an ethnic minority, it was decided to approach those who were liked, trusted and respected within the various communities to help us to locate potential contributors, in order to allay any possible suspicion and mistrust.

The total number of participants in the research was 150. Thirty-one of the individual interviewees had earlier also participated in focus groups. In terms of ethnicity, the numbers break down as shown in the tables below:

Focus Group Details

Ethnicity	Numbers involved
African-Caribbean	34
Asian	43
White non-migrant	18
Polish	26
TOTAL	121

Individual Interviews

Ethnicity	Numbers involved
African-Caribbean	14
Asian	21
White non-migrant	18
Polish	6
Irish	1
TOTAL	60

The above ethnic groupings, however, also consisted of the following subgroups. The African-Caribbean category included first-generation migrants from the Commonwealth of Dominica, Jamaica, Barbados and Trinidad. Those from Dominica were mainly Catholic, while the others were mainly Protestant. The Asian group included first-generation migrants from India, Pakistan and Bangladesh. Some of the Indian and Pakistani women had come to the UK via East Africa. The Pakistani and Bangladeshi participants were all Muslims, while the Indian participants who were Gujarati or Punjabi were Hindus and Sikhs in terms of faith. The Polish women were all Catholics and the non-migrant white women came from both Catholic and different kinds of Protestant backgrounds. The Irish participant was Catholic.

All the minority ethnic women had at some time been married, although many were now widowed and a couple were divorced. The only never married women were in the white non-migrant group. A range of occupations and economic participation rates is represented, although a majority of the Asian women had never been in paid employment. The research covered rural, suburban and inner-city areas.

It had always been our intention to give feedback to our participants. We issued two interim reports, which went to all involved in the research. A final report was sent at the conclusion of our study. We also invited the participants to attend a day meeting in York, as had been promised during the fieldwork. One hundred and forty people attended, a significant proportion of whom were research participants, although some of the gatekeepers who had helped also came, brought to York in hired coaches. Preliminary findings were presented, together with an opportunity for respondents to have further input and discussion of these issues collectively, which some of them did through interpreters. A tour of the City of York was arranged during the afternoon. All this raises the matter of how properly to provide recompense for those who take part in research – itself an under-researched area (Arksey and Knight 1999).

Women in later life: exploring 'race' and ethnicity

Broadly speaking, the women in the research focused on eight major aspects of their lives and experiences to reach conclusions, in their terms, on quality of life. These can be organized in relation to two main themes. The first of these involves physical and material factors. Here the women discussed such matters as their health and issues of embodiment. They reflected on leisure and work opportunities and activities. They also spoke about resources; for example, about money and about access to reasonable housing and transport. There was also a concern about environmental issues, for those who lived in inner cities, for instance, accumulations of rubbish, fear of crime and lack of safety.

The second theme focused on emotional issues, psychological well-being and social support. Here the women concentrated on the benefits of social networks of family and kin, friends and community. The minority ethnic contributors emphasized the significance of shared identities, language, culture and tradition in their lives. The women discussed the role of faith and spirituality throughout the life course, but particularly in relation to aging. They also indicated that bereavement and dying and, for those who were widows, the loss of a partner, were important influences.

Income, although an issue for those who participated in this study, did not emerge as the most central in terms of quality of life. A range of incomes was represented. Although some women worried a lot about the ability to pay bills and were unable to afford many luxuries, most did not report this in terms of having a significant quality of life effect. Although income may be enabling, and more of it would have been welcomed, generally money was not at the top of the agenda.

Health, however, was viewed as *the* most important issue in relation to quality of life, as other researchers have found (Butt and Moriarty 2005; Nazroo et al. 2005). Despite having a range of health-related issues, the majority of our respondents reported getting on with their lives. When interests were under threat due to health problems, participants spoke of their attempts to maintain those interests and to keep active at all costs. This was across the board and many respondents were active contributors to their neighbourhoods and communities.

Although the focus of the research was quality of life and this theme clearly resonates throughout the book, the latter is not concerned with quality of life *per se*. Because we were speaking to women from a range of cultural groups, it seemed important to let the structure and content of the book emerge from what appeared important to them in terms of their own lives. Since the minority ethnic women were migrants, this, along with other life course experiences *as migrants*, was centrally important to them. The significance of family and networks was similarly seen as crucial. Because our respondents themselves identified their health as being so critical, it is necessary to explore what this means to them. Religion and spirituality also emerged as central topics, as did views about death and about widowhood. These then are the areas about which we have chosen to write. The structure of the book is as follows.

In Chapter 2, we look at existing research on older women, focusing, particularly, on income and pensions, health and housing. The fact that the more negative aspects of older women's lives get the most attention is noted, together with the absence of material on minority ethnic older people in general, and older women in particular.

Chapter 3 considers issues of theory and methodology in relation to studying older women. It starts off with an overview of theories and theorizing in social gerontology before going on to consider feminist perspectives on gender and aging. It then looks at issues in relation to ethnicity and aging, particularly the argument that sometimes the theoretical and conceptual frameworks that have been developed by later life researchers are inappropriate for use in different cultural contexts. The chapter explores what we call a post-gerontology approach, one that attempts to go beyond taken-for-granted assumptions about theory's cultural neutrality. It uses ideas about empowerment and disempowerment to do this, before ending with a brief discussion about some methodological research issues that have arisen from our work.

In Chapter 4, we look at the meaning of identity and life course events for the women in our study. The chapter begins by considering participants' views about when they became 'old' if, indeed, they believe they have, and how they perceive they are regarded as an older person. It moves on to explore issues of ethnicity, nationality and identification, specifically how the women see themselves in relation to place of birth, cultural background and current nationality. The chapter explores women's wartime experiences, the migration process and the latter's legacy, illustrating some of the truly dreadful times our participants have been through. This leads on to a discussion of the early racism experienced, especially, by the African-Caribbean women. The chapter finishes by looking at the contributors' views about employment and retirement. These are significant in terms of what has occurred over the life course and how the memories still resonate today.

Chapter 5 focuses on family, networks and what we refer to as the moral economy of kin. It first looks at ideas about dependence, independence, interdependence and autonomy and what the idea of a moral economy might mean. It then examines the overwhelming significance of family and kin for the women, across all ethnic groups in this study, before focusing on what this means for the moral economy of kin *per se*. Here notions of duty, obligation and reciprocity are central. The chapter considers next the experience of grandmothering. This is treated to a section on its own, because although part of the moral economy of kin, it is also additionally seen as a deep source of joy, happiness and satisfaction. Being a grandmother was regarded as an achievement, not just in the sense of creating a new role but also as a new aspect of identity. The chapter ends with a look at the ways in which for those mainly more affluent and rural-based women, who do not have proximate family, friendship networks can become an alternative substitute for kin.

The focus in Chapter 6 is on our contributors' views on health and well-being. Its aim is to contest the ways in which uncritical Western and medicalized notions of health are applied to older women. It begins by looking at current theoretical approaches to studying health and well-being before outlining participants' views on the importance of health and the meanings attached to it. The chapter goes on to consider the impact of previous life events on health and then focuses on the body, particularly the significance attached to changes in agility and mobility during aging. It concludes by arguing that there is a need to develop approaches to health and aging that are sensitive to cultural diversity and ethnicity.

Chapter 7 examines religion, faith and spirituality, resources that are often ignored for older people and which are, therefore, under-researched. It aims to demonstrate how the women in our research used these resources and, across ethnic groupings, valued them. The first part of the chapter offers an introduction to current debates about the nature of religion in contemporary society. It then explores the importance of religion for the women in our study, how for many it is part of their identity and sense of self, how they have reflexively personalized their religion and the significance of spirituality in relation to this. The chapter goes on to explore, on the one hand, some of the social benefits contributors clearly gained via their religious involvement before considering, on the other hand, some of the difficulties, for both formal and informal worship, that aging brings, as well as the issue of doubt.

Chapter 8 is concerned with death and dying. A context relating to current debates about attitudes to the latter is provided first, including some details about how dying is viewed in different religions. The chapter then moves on to explore participants' experiences of bereavement across the life course. It next examines women's views about their own death, finding that they are quite fatalistic about the event itself and more concerned about the processes that might lead up to it. The remainder of the chapter considers the death of a husband/partner and the experiences of widowhood. This had come as a shocking and harrowing rite of passage to the women to whom we talked.

In Chapter 9, Conclusions, we briefly discuss the contribution of the book to understanding the relationships between age, gender and ethnicity and situate our study in terms of the life history approach.

Overall, this text aims to make a contribution to understanding what is important in older women's lives across a range of ethnic groups. As Finch says in the Foreword to the book, *Women and aging*, 'Older people are of increasing importance to the vitality, stability and development of this society. Women are crucial to these' (2000: xv).

2

The lives of older women

Introduction

Older people tend to be a relatively disadvantaged group in British society. This is also influenced by factors such as social class and previous occupational status. It is also the case that significant inequalities exist between men and women in the older age groups. These inequities stem mainly, although not entirely, from the fact that the latter are in receipt of lower incomes. Ginn, Street and Arber have noted that older women are more than twice as likely to live in poverty as men (2001). They are also more likely to have higher levels of disability and to experience chronic (that is persistent as opposed to acute) illnesses. Older women are also more likely to live in poor housing stock and to have difficulties with such things as adequate heating and maintenance of buildings. As a consequence, research indicates that finance/income, health and housing form an important basis for older women's material disadvantage (Maynard 1999). Transport and social mobility generally are also important. All these elements relate together in ways that can enhance or debilitate positive effects in the others. Overlying them are aegist views and cultural stereotyping of older people, which are particularly deprecating and demeaning of older women.

This chapter is concerned with what is currently known about older women's experiences of later life. It is impossible in one chapter to document this down to the finest detail. Instead, what are deemed to be the most significant and salient aspects are discussed. The chapter begins by discussing what is understood by the phrase 'being older' and looks at the socially constructed nature of the idea of 'old age'. It then considers the financial implications of later life for women, particularly their lesser entitlement to and access to pensions when compared to men. Following this, the focus is on gender and women's health in the context where the latter is seen as being particularly significant for older people. The chapter then moves on to explore housing and living arrangements, before also focusing on transport and mobility issues more generally. Finally, the chapter considers some of the positive aspects of the aging process for women before concluding with some general remarks.

What is meant by being older?

Age is a socially constructed category. It also differs culturally and historically (Wilson 2000; Thane 2002; Vincent 2003). In Western cultures chronological age, a person's age in years, is usually considered to be most important because it is used to determine when individuals can engage in certain activities, for example consensual sex, and their eligibility for particular state and welfare benefits, for instance the state pension. However, other ways of talking about age are sometimes added to this. Physiological age, for instance, refers to the physical transformations an individual experiences over time, for older people such things as greying hair or the appearance of wrinkles. Social age relates to what are deemed to be the appropriate attitudes and behaviours for a particular age group. This is also connected to a person's subjective perceptions of themselves; that is how old they feel or see themselves to be, along with ascribed age, how the person thinks they are seen by others. For women, of course, the latter can be particularly important. As Sontag famously claimed, 'Getting older is less profoundly wounding for a man ... Men are "allowed" to age, without penalty, in several ways that women are not' (1978: 73). The aging female is, generally, regarded as not attractive, whereas different standards hold for the aging male. Women are heavily pressurized to keep themselves looking young and this is regarded as being less important for men (Featherstone and Hepworth 2000). However, overall, the point is that these three ways of looking at aging, the chronological, the physiological and the social, cannot be inferred from each other. There is no necessary interdependence between where individuals are located on one and where they are positioned in rela-

14

tion to the others. It is agist to assume that people will have particular
needs, attitudes, behaviours or disabilities simply on the basis of their
age.

If ideas about age and aging provoke difficulties, there are similar
problems when it comes to defining later life itself. Commentators
differ as to how it should be defined and, in many ways, the issue is
becoming increasingly problematic as the boundaries between stages of
life, in relation to chronology, become increasingly fluid (Gilleard and
Higgs 2000). This can be seen in the fact that more women work into
their late 50s and more men are retiring before the statutory retirement
age (Ginn, Street and Arber 2001). Arber and Ginn point out that the
two main social markers of later life in western societies, men's
retirement and widowhood, have moved in opposite directions during
the 20th century (1991). The former have tended to occur earlier and
the latter later in life. Further, due to increases in longevity, many argue
that it is necessary to demarcate phases within people's later years. A
distinction between the young-old and the old-old is now routinely
made, with the categories usually referring to the 60–74 and 75 plus age
groups respectively. Others differentiate between what are called the
third and the fourth ages, although some object to the assumed
homogeneity in these terms, arguing that the fourth age, seen as time of
greater dependency, has merely taken over from how the third age used
to be seen (Gilleard and Higgs 2000).

Despite all this, however, although there is some arbitrariness in
selecting a specific age as marking the start of later life, most
researchers and policy-makers in Britain see retirement as its symbolic
beginning. This poses problems of comparability since currently in
Britain, this is different for men and women, with the former being
able to draw their state pension from 65 years, whereas women can do
so from the age of 60. A phased process of 'equalization', whereby
women's retirement age will be brought in line with men's will begin in
April 2010. However, the issues of retirement and pensions are particular thorny ones for women. It is to these that the chapter now turns.

The pension problem for women

The capacity to secure an independent income in one's own right is a
critical aspect of gender equality. Yet, men and women are not equal in

this regard. Pension policy-making in Britain has been characterized by instability and uncertainty. There have been marked changes of direction at regular intervals and these have had particular consequences for women (Evason and Spence 2002). It has been pointed out that women have been largely invisible in the debate about pensions and that their interests and the challenges posed by their different patterns of life have rarely been considered. This might be regarded as strange given, as has already been seen in the Introduction, that the majority of pensioners are, in fact, women (Evason and Spence 2002).

The difficulties that women have in securing adequate pensions arise from the gendered roles they play and the experiences they have throughout the life course. A gendered division of labour means that such factors as family caring commitments, unpaid domestic work, lower pay, proclivity for part-time employment and the so-called 'career-breaks' at the birth of children all leave women with lower lifetime earnings when compared to men (Ginn, Daly and Street 2001). Further, current government policy, which increases reliance on private pension schemes, thereby reducing what can be expected from state provision, is likely to perpetuate the disadvantages that older women currently face and these look likely to be projected into the future (Ginn 2003). This is because such a policy is built upon a male model that is assumed to be able to maintain full employment throughout the working life. This is something that is difficult for many women and was certainly not the norm for the current older female generation in the past (Ginn, 2003; Ginn, Daly and Street 2001). Until recently, many pension schemes have been based on assumptions concerning women's dependence on a male breadwinner. Further, women generally are also less likely to be involved in private or occupational pension schemes. Although savings and investments are also important influences on economic status, these are also areas where women are under-represented. It is mainly an individual's employment career, together with that of any spouse or partner, which is a significant determinant of income in later life. Women's opportunities have been far more restricted than men's in the past and inequalities and double standards still remain.

The Equal Opportunities Commission (EOC) report (2007), *Completing the Revolution*, indicates that women's retirement income is 40

16

percent less than men's and predicts that at the current rate of progress it will take 45 years to eradicate this 'pensions gap'. Further, its gender equality index shows that, in relation to those factors identified as increasing the likelihood of pension famine, progress is either painfully slow or non-existent. Drawing on government statistics, the index suggests, for instance, that it will take 20 years to equalize men and women's full-time hourly pay and 25 years for female part-time hourly rates to reach those of full-time males. There has been no change in the gender segregation of occupations, so that 65 percent of all occupational groups are dominated by either men or women. Although the situation regarding child care is improving, with men taking on more of this activity, that with regard to other forms of domestic work seems to be worsening. Time use surveys indicate that women spend 78 percent more time per day on housework than men (Lader et al. 2006). The EOC concludes that unless something is done to change these gender divisions, 'our children's children will still be grappling with the same challenges' in the future (EOC 2007: 1).

The fact that women pensioners are relatively poor has been confirmed in a recent government report. This noted that only 23 percent of them were receiving a full state pension and only 17 percent of them in relation to their own contributions record (Department of Work and Pensions 2005). This is because from 1948 until 1977 women who were married paid a reduced rate of National Insurance, called the married women's stamp. This entitled them to virtually nothing and did not bequeath rights to a pension in their own right. Instead, women who paid this stamp, as most of them did, had to rely on their husband's contributions record and wait until he reached 65 years of age (Ginn, Street and Arber 2001). The woman would then receive 60 percent of her husband's pension. If the man was under retirement age, it was assumed that he was working and that he would support his wife on his earnings. Not only are many of today's older women's lack of pensions due to these archaic rules, a married woman who was paying the reduced rate at the time that it was abolished was allowed to carry on doing so as long as she did so continuously. Around 100 000 married women who are currently working still make this anachronistic payment and it is estimated that more than one million women under 60 have paid it at some time (DWP 2005). Despite the introduction of Home Responsibilities Protection in 1978 (which protects

the basic state pension record for men and women who have significant long-term care responsibilities) and Pension Credit in 2003 (a
means-tested top-up for those below a certain income level), older
women are still destined to have to manage on low incomes during
their later years. The DWP (2005) estimates that two-thirds of people
in receipt of pension credit, because their incomes are so low, are
women and half of these are aged 75 or over.

A further factor in this somewhat complicated equation is that many
older people, particularly women, fail to take up the array of means
tested benefits for which they are eligible. (Brewer et al. 2007). This is
due to the fact that people do not know about their existence, they
resent the intrusive questions that means-testing implies, and they find
it difficult to access the forms and even more difficult to follow the
bureaucracy to complete them (Craig et al. 2003). It has been suggested
that automatic payment of benefits might help to ameliorate these
problems.

Information about the experiences of older minority ethnic women
in relation to income and pensions is not particularly easy to obtain. In
the recent DWP (2005) report on women and pensions, for example, it
is noticeable that the chapter on 'the ethnic minority dimension' is the
shortest of all at just over ten pages . The research that does exist
indicates that in, general, older people from minority ethnic groups are
at increased risk of economic disadvantage, when compared to their
white counterparts (Ginn and Arber 2000; Berthoud 2002; Butt and
Moriarty 2005; Nazroo et al. 2005). For instance, in Nazroo et al.'s
(2005) analysis of inequalities between different ethnic groups in later
life, it was found that the greatest discrepancy between the latter and
white older people was in levels of income. However, it was also noted
that elderly people from minority ethnic groups do not uniquely
experience income inequalities, nor are they uniformly faced. Much
diversity was found to exist within individual groupings. This was
supported by Berthoud (2002) in his research which showed that,
although those of Indian and African-Caribbean origin were poorer
than the white population, their income was well above that of those
from the Bangladeshi and Pakistani population who were very poor
indeed. The Chinese had the highest income of all groups, including
the white category. Evandrou (2000) has also reported similar findings
for older people from minority ethnic groups.

Whereas African-Caribbean and Indian women as a whole have economic activity rates approaching those of the white population, those of the Pakistani and Bangladeshi groups are relatively low (Ginn and Arber 2000; DWP 2005). This is due to cultural traditions but it also limits their capacity to accumulate pension provisions or savings to support them in later life. While these women are part of the generation that expected to be cared for by family and kin, especially sons, research does suggest, as with the findings of our study reported elsewhere in this book, a degree of ambivalence in relation to this (Katbamna, 2004; Barnes and Taylor 2006). Participants in Katbamna's study, which included Gujarati and Bangladeshi males and females, reported that, although they felt that they were morally entitled to claim support from their children, they might not choose to do this. There is also some evidence that South Asian women are less likely to control their own finances than other groups (Barnard and Pettigrew 2003). Given their lack of employment history, this could place the women in a difficult situation.

Research has also suggested that those from minority ethnic communities are also under-pensioned and less likely to have a private pension when compared to the white population (Pensions Policy Institute 2003; DWP 2005). Indeed, both Barnes and Taylor (2006) and Katbamna (2004) indicate a lack of awareness, information and forethought about retirement and pensions in the respondents to whom they spoke. It seems likely that, for those minority women who are working, their pension situation will be similar to that of the white women described above. However, given that they tend to earn even less than the latter and with the possibility of unexpected life events, it is probable that they are in an even more vulnerable position.

Similarly, Barnard and Pettigrew cite ignorance about the benefits system and lack of knowledge about eligibility as major reasons for minority ethnic people not making a claim (2003). Language barriers can exacerbate this problem, particularly for women and one study found that older women of South Asian origin were particularly confused about procedures (Craig et al. 2003). There was also a prevalent apprehension among older minority ethnic people, some of whom were frightened of making a claim lest it should lead to an investigation of their children, loss of savings or income or a challenge to their residency status (Barnard and Pettigrew 2003). It is likely that minority ethnic women are more prone to such views than men, with a corresponding effect on their income.

Thus, women from minority groups potentially face multiple economic disadvantages in later life (DWP 2005). In addition to the gender pay gap issues, which affect all women regardless of ethnicity, they share the discrimination and disadvantages encountered by such communities as a whole. The economic inequalities that affect them today derive from previous migration patterns and employment opportunities, since upon their arrival here there was an unequal distribution of workers into low-paid employment (Patel 1999). Racism was also prevalent during their working lives in terms of levels of pay and restricting job progression. With regard to pensions, with the exception of the African-Caribbean group, women from ethnic minorities are less likely than those who are white to be eligible for the state pension. The DWP (2005) figures indicate that, even when they are receiving the state pension, it is more likely to be the basic one only and will not include the second state pension, which exists as a form of safety net.

The significance of health

Health features very highly in older people's own measures of quality of life and this is the case for both men and women and across ethnic groups (Siddell 1995; Smith 2000; McMunn et al. 2005). It was also the case for the participants in our study, as discussed in the Introduction and in Chapter 6. However, in the past there have been a number of problems when considering health issues and older people because this tended to focus on the presence, absence or indicators of disease. This has led commentators to point out that focusing centrally on morbidity as indicative of health can be both negative and patronizing (Arber and Cooper 2000). It takes no account of people's subjective feelings, their individual capacities and contributes to the view that later life is a time of decrepitude, dependency and a drain on resources. Further, it fails to recognize that many older people, and indeed older women, are not infirm or in ill-health. The difficulty here is one of dealing simultaneously with two separate issues. On the one hand, there is the need to counter agist stereotypes. On the other, there is an obligation not to minimize the real health problems that exist for some people and their need for sensitive and coordinated health services. For instance, older women are particularly prone to conditions that are not life-threatening but remain highly symptomatic and for which there is usually no cure. Many more women than men have arthritis, for example, and the percentage increases with age, whereas it decreases for men (Arber 1998; Arber and Cooper 1999). Siddell comments that this pattern between the sexes reflects a general trend for many chronic illnesses (Siddell 1995). While it is the case that long-standing illnesses do not necessarily imply disability or immobility, they can lead to degrees of incapacity. Older women are also more likely to suffer fractures. This is due both to osteoporosis and to their higher incidence of falling, which are linked, it is suggested, to such things as hypothermia, drugs that induce dizziness and the over-prescribing of tranquillizers (Siddell 1993). Thus, although the vast majority of people in later life are able to do such tasks as care for themselves, shop and move around outside the home, women are more likely to be incapacitated than men (Arber and Cooper 2000). Those over 65 years old are more than twice as likely as men to report impaired mobility, with the very elderly being severely affected (Arber 1998). Given the increased possibility that such women will be living on their own, one consequence is that they are likely to require enhanced informal and statutory care.

Another difficulty faced by those in later life is the commonly held view that aging involves a steady and largely inevitable deterioration in physical and mental abilities. Professional workers may be particularly prone to this kind of negative view, since they normally meet mainly those who are frail and infirm (Graham 2000). As a consequence, older people, and older women in particular, often experience difficulties with the kind of information they are given and the agist ways in which they are treated when seeking advice on health issues. Siddell (1993) refers to research in which older women objected to their GPs' frequent diagnoses that their condition was a reflection of their age, rather than any other factors. Many older women in her study felt that they were made to feel guilty about visiting a doctor and had extremely low expectations about obtaining relief for their symptoms. The women felt that they were hardly listened to and that their doctors paid scant attention to their version of things, preferring instead to offer a prescription rather than engaging in a more lengthy consultation (Siddell

1993; Bernard 2000). This is also supported by other findings (Doyal et al. 1998).

Although there are some notable exceptions, it is not particularly easy to find out about the specific health needs and patterns of older minority ethnic women outside of those that look at this in strictly epidemiological terms (Cooper and Arber 2003). This is because most researchers work on either gender or ethnicity but not so often on both. Government statistics indicate that, overall, Pakistani women followed by those from Bangladesh report the highest levels of poor health with Indian and African-Caribbean women coming next (National Statistics 2001). People of Chinese origin claimed the lowest rates of ill-health, the incidence of which was roughly equal across gender, lower than those of the white group. Similarly, more Pakistani and Bangladeshi women reported having a long-term illness or disability that restricted their daily activity rates than any other group, including the white category, although it has to be said that the rate for men was also high. Again, the Chinese respondents had the lowest rate of restriction.

It has been pointed out that inequalities present throughout the life course increase with age (Nazroo 2004). Thus, it is to be expected that the trends reported here will be exacerbated as people get older. Indeed, Butt and Moriarty (2005) and Nazroo et al. (2005) have reported on the significant health problems of the older people in their studies, particularly those from the Asian communities. There is a clear association between factors such as low income, poor housing and ethnicity. Research also indicates that socio-economic deprivation can lead to poor health (Ginn and Arber 2000; Office of the Deputy Prime Minister 2003).

There is also evidence that, while people from minority ethnic groups are the heaviest users of primary care services, they often receive inadequate treatment and fail to get access to adequate services (Age Concern 2002). This is a particular issue for Bangladeshi and Pakistani older women for whom culture, custom and language difficulties can play a significant part in their under-referral to secondary health care. Other problems, such as insensitive dietary provision or failure to meet preference for same gender carers and service providers may also inhibit some women's contact with the health services (Lowdell et al. 2000).

Housing and other issues

Living arrangements are another factor that can exacerbate or minimize the financial and physical effects of advancing years and housing
has been identified as a key dimension to quality of life and well being
(Heywood et al. 2002), Contrary to some of the stereotypes, only about
5 percent of those over 65 years old live in residential homes, with the
majority being in the 75 plus year group and, therefore, women. This
means, however, that most of the remaining 95 percent of older people
largely fend for themselves (ONS 2002). Approximately 90 percent of
older people live in either owner-occupied or publically or privately
rented accommodation. The remaining 5 percent live in some form of
sheltered housing (ONS 2002). This is a purpose-built form of
accommodation aimed at elderly people who are less able-bodied but
who still wish to maintain independent living. The demographic trends
of increased longevity and widowhood mean that this form of housing
is more likely to be occupied by women. Further, the 2001 Census
shows that there has been a 30 percent increase in single person
households over a decade (ONS 2002). Nearly half of all such households (3.1 million) are pensioners and nearly three quarters of these are
older women (2.4 million).

The tenure patterns of the older population are usually the result of
housing choices made in the past, when the housing market was rather
different to how it is today. The private rented sector, in particular, was
more important and currently older people are more likely to be in
rented accommodation generally and less likely to be home owners
when compared to the rest of the population (Age Concern 2002).
However, low income lies at the root of older people's concerns about
housing and this is particularly problematic for women. As Arber and
Ginn remark, 'balancing a fear of high heating bills against the discomfort of cold and damp is a dilemma common to tenants and
owners' (1991: 103). Further, women who are widowed may have
trouble in maintaining their houses. In 2004, for example, there were
some three million households with at least one person aged 60 or over
which were classified as non-decent. This comprised 37 percent of all
such homes. Of these 676 000 of the oldest occupants are aged 75–84
and a further 232 000 are 85 or over (Department for Communities
and Local Government 2006). Where women are still living in the

family home, there are also issues regarding its size and compatibility with solo life (Heywood et al. 2002). However, this also has to be balanced against notions of what the house means to them, its memories and associations and feelings of home. While moving may appear a more realistic option to outsiders, particularly since older housing stock is more difficult to adapt, this may not seem to be a possible choice from the point of view of older women themselves (Gurney and Means 1993).

In addition, if they are home owners, older people in general and widows in particular may find themselves to be 'equity rich' but 'income poor'. This refers to their inability to realize the capital contained in the bricks and mortar of their home without selling it, and the subsequent reliance of many on state benefits for a weekly income. The presence of steps and stairs in a house may also present an obstacle to independent living. Yet, the policies of governments in Britain, particularly in the 1980s, in encouraging home ownership have severely restricted the ability of local authorities to build new public housing of any kind. As Arber and Ginn (1991) point out, this has especially affected the supply of sheltered housing, which is attractive to many older women because it may offer a degree of social and physical support, safety and security. Instead, the private sector is increasingly taking over the provision of retirement appartments and sheltered housing for sale. While this may be attractive to affluent couples, it is beyond the means of most elderly women.

Minority ethnic older women, of course, are likely to face the same housing issues as their white counterparts. However, the whole area of the housing aspirations and expectations of older people from minority ethnic communities has been largely unexplored and there appears to be virtually nothing on older women *per se* (ODPM 2003). For minority ethnic groups in general levels of unemployment, low incomes and discrimination all mean that finding accommodation may not be easy (Somerville and Steele 2001). There is also a tendency to cluster geographically together with people from similar backgrounds and these groups also tend to reside in less popular inner-city areas. While this is not necessarily problematic, it is the continuing association between this segregation and deprivation that is the issue. Harassment from landlords, neighbours and other local people in some areas can also create difficulties. Somerville and Steele's (2001) work has shown how racism affects the housing choices available to black and other minority groups and how this contributes to their social exclusion. There has been criticism of the effectiveness of responses to racist harassment and the lack of implementation by official bodies, including social housing landlords, of good practices to counter it (ODPM, 2003). There is also evidence that minority ethnic groups disproportionately face other housing problems. People of Pakistani and Bangladeshi origin, for instance, are particularly disadvantaged compared to those who are white, since they are less likely to be owner-occupiers and much more likely to live in overcrowded, poor-quality housing and to be dissatisfied with it (ODPM 2003; Garvie 2004). African-Caribbean people are also relatively disadvantaged, although less so than the Pakistanis and the Bangladeshis, and they are at least more likely to be owner-occupiers.

Thus, while research gives some indication of the situation of minority ethnic groups with regard to housing, there is much more to be done. The needs of older people and of older women need to brought more centrally into the frame. One area that requires consideration, given the projected figures for increasing numbers of the elderly and some evidence of the beginning breakdown of three generational living in the Asian community, is the culturally and religiously sensitive provision of residential and nursing care (Patel 1999).

The financial, health and housing difficulties experienced by women in later life also relate to other aspects of their material circumstances. Of particular importance is transport. Older women are less likely to own or drive a car than older men and are, therefore, more reliant on public transport. This is particularly the case for minority ethnic women. However, as state subsidies for public transport have been cut, so the services provided have become less user-friendly, from the point of view of older women across all groups. For instance, bus timetables have been reduced and the elimination of bus conductors, train guards and station personnel on many services decreases the perceived efficiency and safety of what is being provided (Gilhooly et al. 1999; Maynard 1999). Yet, many older women depend on public transport for maintaining social networks and for activities such as shopping (Holland et al. 2005). This is particularly so if they live on remote housing estates or in areas far removed from out-of-town shopping complexes (Arber and Ginn 1991). Reliance on local retailers often makes purchases much more costly. Even when public transport is more readily available, older people may be discouraged from making use of the facility. Problems of climbing into buses and trains, having to stand in crushed and crowded conditions, and automatically closing doors, which may catch clothes or even limbs, all add to the perceived hazards of travelling (Maynard 1999). Gilhooly et al. (2003) report from their study on later life, which included both men and women, that 28 potential barriers to using public transport were identified by them. Concern was most expressed about personal security, with 65 percent of participants voicing worries about this if travelling during the evening or at night.

Transport difficulties, however, are only one aspect of the more general mobility problems that older women may experience. Independent living is not necessarily easy if there are steps and stairs to countenance at home or a kitchen that is not designed compactly and for efficient use. Access to the local community can also be restricted by buildings that lack ramps or lifts, congested roads and pavements and poor provision of activities that are likely to attract older people and encourage them into social and collective environments (Maynard 1999). All these things are particularly significant for older women of all ethnic groups, when so many live on their own. Thus, potential isolation, and possible loneliness, compound the other material disadvantages with which they are faced.

Living through and with aging

So far this chapter has considered some of the disadvantages and inequalities associated with later life, the differences that exist between men and women and how these might relate to the experiences of those from minority ethnic groups. However, although a lot of the research and literature concentrates on these negative aspects, more work is beginning to emerge that looks at the processes of aging in more positive ways. While not denying the difficulties that exist for some, this shows that the later years can be both rewarding and enjoyable. Aging should not be seen as some kind of a condition that requires inevitable treatment by doctors, social workers and other professionals or as some final stage with which an individual has to cope. Rather, women and men live *through* and *with* aging. This involves the possible opening up of new experiences, with the connotation that later life is not some kind of end state but a time when old pleasures can be enjoyed as well as new ones created. This can be particularly positive for women. As one respondent to research on widowhood exclaimed, as a result of reflecting on life since the death of her husband and the new pursuits followed, 'I've surprised myself, I suppose ...' (Maynard 1998). While bereavement necessarily involves grief and feelings of loss, as is graphically described in Chapter 7, widowhood can lead to new freedoms and opportunities, with new roles sometimes becoming available (Chambers 2005).

For instance, for some older women later life brings the opportunity of increased freedom to travel and involvement in leisure and other pursuits, although the image of 'older people as jet-setting hedonists, pursuing pleasure around the globe is ... only applicable to a minority' (Jarvis et al. 1996: 20). However, the opposite picture of older people as too poor to have leisure activities is also misleading. Despite the difficulties of defining leisure in this context (one person's form of enjoyment may be another's *bête noire*), it is clear that not all such pursuits need to be costly. While participation in both indoor and outdoor pastimes does decline with age (notable exceptions being gardening and walking), some activities remain at a fairly constant level (Bernard and Meade 1993; Richards 2005). For older women, across ethnic groups, these are predominantly home-based and domestic, involving watching television, visiting and entertaining friends, reading, needlework and knitting (Maynard 1999).

Another activity with which older women are involved is voluntary work, although this applies more to those from the middle classes. Volunteering may include fund-raising, work in charity shops, visiting those in hospital or residential homes and offering practical help in the home. Around 30 percent of older women also join clubs. However, only 13 percent seem to go to those that cater only for older people and these generally seem more attractive to those from the working class (Bernard and Meade 1993; Scott and Wenger 1995). Older women, and particularly those from black and minority ethnic groups, are also involved in religious-based, church and community activities, as is described in later chapters of this book.

A significant factor in older women's ability to live through aging is the existence of social and support networks (Jerrome 1993a, b; de Jong Gierveld 2003; Davidson et al. 2005). Evidence suggests that they have on average more friends than men and that the quality of their relationships also differs. While women's female friends are often close confidantes, men tend to rely on their wives to fulfil this function (Scott and Wenger 1995). Whereas men's work-based friendships may be broken or weakened on retirement, women are more likely to replace lost friendships and to continue to make new friends throughout the life course. As a result, it has been suggested that older women may have a psychological, emotional and social advantage over their male counterparts (Jerrome 1993b; Scott and Wenger 1995). Arber and Ginn claim, for example, that 'although elderly women's opportunities for making and maintaining friendships are constrained by lack of material and health resources relative to elderly men's, their relationship skills acquired in early life are an asset. They are less likely than their husbands to have placed all their emotional 'eggs in one basket' and seem more adaptable to changed circumstances' (1991: 169). Arber and Ginn go on to add that friendships can help to alleviate the effects of older women's disadvantages in material and health resources. Often embedded in a network of women friends with shared interests, such friendships provide a basis for a variety of joint activities, from shopping and local outings to travel and holidays. This is highly important in a society that values feminine youth and heterosexual coupledom, often making social life difficult for older women who are on their own. Strong and positive friendship groups provide a way of fighting back and a means through which they can re-enter social and community life (Chambers 2005).

Conclusion

This chapter has reviewed research that looks at some of the main ways in which older women experience disadvantage and inequality. In this it has only been possible to consider areas that have been given major consideration in the literature. However, it is clear that income, health and housing have been seen as significant mediators in women's later life experiences. In particular, the gendered nature of pension policy and provision is increasingly a cause for concern. However, while older women's experiences and the nature of gender issues are beginning to be explored in greater depth, the significance of ethnicity in relation to later life and, especially the implications of this for women, are very under-explored. Further, the conceptual underpinning to all this is very underdeveloped. It is, therefore, to issues about the theoretical frameworks that are the basis of studying later life and the extent to which they might be seen to be culturally loaded to which we now turn.

3

Studying older women: issues of theory and methodology

Introduction

In the preface to their text, *Handbook on Theories of Aging*, Bengtson and Schaie (1999) argue that there is a need to re-establish the significance of theory in exploring later life. While empirical research on the lives of older people has been increasing, this has tended to focus on issues of needs, welfare and social care provision. Such work has mainly involved describing the problems and experiences of later life, rather than making connections between aging and social, political, cultural and other systems (Estes 1979). Bengston and Schaie challenge the idea, articulated by empiricists and postmodernists alike, that theory is 'outmoded' or 'little more than intellectual nonsense' (1999: ix). Predicting that the first years of the 21st century will bring 'an avalanche in research publications reporting data about problems and processes of aging', they express the hope that writers will 'also address the theoretical implications of their findings', with a view to providing better explanations (1999: x). They see the role of theory as a way of accounting for and understanding the nature of the empirical data.

Similar views about the relation of theory to later life research have been put forward by other writers. Estes et al. (2003) for example, also support the exhortation for theory to be more articulated with the results of empirical studies, suggesting that it is the lack of a relationship between the two, rather than the lack of theory *per se* that is the issue. However, despite the fact that a number of commentators have attempted to put theoretical issues in relation to later life onto the intellectual agenda (the work of those such as Estes 1979, 2001; Cole 1992; Moody 1993; Holstein and Gubrium 2000; Biggs et al. 2003), for example, spring readily to mind), the subject remains largely, as Birren once remarked, 'data rich and theory poor' (Birren and Bengston 1988).

There have also been challenges to researching later life on the methodological front. Traditionally, the tendency was mainly to focus on quantitative research, with an emphasis on producing statistical generalizations, facts and figures. However, the benefits of in-depth qualitative research are now more generally appreciated. In particular, the significance of a life history approach, of the autobiographical method and of reminiscence and memory research is being emphasized, along with the more obvious interviewing and focus group formats (Jamieson and Victor 2002). The role that older people themselves might play in the research process is also increasingly being recognized, with some commentators questioning the ethics and propriety of doing research 'on' older subjects (Cook et al. 2004). Qualitative research, with its emphasis on understanding the social world from the point of view of research participants themselves, is then now an accepted and legitimate way of researching older people.

The purpose of this chapter is to examine some of the current theoretical and methodological issues being discussed in social gerontology. The intention is to provide a general overview of some trends, as well as providing a contextual framework for the rest of the book. The chapter begins by offering a background to the study of women and aging. It does this by giving a brief history of the theorizing of aging, before moving on to consider how it has portrayed older women and the extent to which ethnic and cultural diversity has been addressed. The chapter draws attention to feminist perspectives on gender and aging, but also points to the neglect of later life work generally to consider ethnic and cultural variation. Drawing on the research that provides the basis for this book, it argues for a 'post'-gerontological framework and for a nuanced use of the concepts of 'empowerment' and 'disempowerment'. This then leads to a briefer discussion of some of the methodological issues that arose from our research on women, ethnicity and later life. The chapter concludes that a greater sensitivity to cultural difference needs to become part of both theoretical and methodological discussions in relation to aging research.

Theorizing aging

Most commentators see social gerontology as developing a specific identity in the 1940s and early 1950s. Informed by the biomedical model of aging, which sees it as the gradual deterioration of both mind and body, most work up until the 1960s focused on physical and social decline and the social problems that later life was increasingly expected to bring. The argument tended to be that growing older is synonymous with decrepitude, poverty, poor housing and a loss of self-autonomy and independence (Posner 1995; Phillipson 1998). In the social sciences, these assumptions were aligned to the theoretical ideas of functionalism, disengagement and role theory. Although each of these adopted slightly different ways of understanding the significance of old age 'decline', the emphasis of them all was on the negative factors associated with aging.

For example, the functionalist approach emphasized how no longer having a positive function to play in society (paid work for men and children, leaving the 'nest' for women) led to a crisis of identity and diminishing self-esteem. Similarly, role theory and disengagement theory are premised on the idea that the 'normal' aging process requires older people to withdraw from previous activities and roles and to 'disengage' from society (Phillipson 1998). From a social structural point of view, they are eased out of roles in which they can no longer function effectively. In individual terms, disengagement enables an older person to conserve limited energy by having a restricted number of roles to perform and associated role partners. Psychologically, there is emotional adjustment and preparation for death. Overall, older people's relatively low social status and lack of social, economic and individual resources mean that they have nothing much of value in terms of social exchange, except as a recipient for past favours. These approaches emphasize how older people adjust to later life following, for example, retirement and widowhood.

With hindsight, of course, it is not difficult to criticize these perspectives for their emphasis on aging as an individual social problem, their lack of attention to people's own meanings and experiences and their failure to move beyond gender stereotyping. Further, there was no acknowledgement that roles might be sustained as well as lost, that there might be relief, rather than distress, at losing them or that there might be re-engagement with previous activities and even engagement with new ones. The idea that disengagement and loss of role or function is a desirable outcome is also ethnocentric and clearly does not resonate with the experiences of those in other cultures at that time. It has also been suggested that these were not so much 'theories' as normative frameworks in which tacit assumptions were being made about what was appropriate socially for those in later life. As Phillipson has pointed out, conventional theorizing in social gerontology came to be seen as 'colluding with a repressive and intolerant society' and its value has been seen more in terms of acting as a spur to argument and debate than as a contribution to explanation or understanding (1998: 16). Nonetheless, although the approaches themselves are in disrepute and social gerontology has been changing rapidly, the biomedical model on which they were based still remains, to some extent, the fulcrum upon which a significant amount of later life research is premised.

During the 1970s later life scholars were introduced to a variety of new theories from a range of sources and disciplines. These included neo-Marxism, neo-Weberianism, neo-Frankfurt School and symbolic interactionism. Attempts were made to move beyond simply focusing at the individual level and develop more macro-level accounts (Estes et al. 2003). However, it is with the development of what is known as critical gerontology, which really took root in the 1980s, that major changes to previous ways of thinking came to be seen. Of particular importance here was the political economy perspective, which still exerts an influence on how commentators explain and make sense of the experiences of later life.

The political economic model emphasizes the socially constructed nature of later life in an attempt directly to challenge the biomedical approach. It was argued that the experiences of aging were influenced by the division of labour and resulting inequalities in advanced capitalist societies, rather than by biological factors (Estes 1979; Townsend 1981; Walker 1981; Phillipson 1982; Estes et al. 1984). Older people were placed in the position of 'structured dependency' due to their forced exclusion from work, brought about by the retirement age, and their consequent experience of poverty and restricted roles. Estes (1979), for example, referred to the 'aging enterprise', pointing out that older people were often treated as commodities and that policies tended to stigmatize and isolate them from the rest of society. The role of the state in managing the relationship between the individual and society and in allocating scarce resources was also emphasized. The political economic model also considered differential experiences of aging, particularly those of class, thereby contesting previously taken-for-granted assumptions about homogeneity.

This perspective has exerted a huge influence on social gerontology and is still being developed by proponents. However, it is not without criticism. For instance, it still retains a largely negative perspective on aging. Despite an emphasis on social divisions, it has only recently begun to pay significant attention to gender and ethnicity, often seeing them only in relation to the economy and the labour market. It has been suggested that the approach is overdeterministic and fails to consider how individuals have agency and may be able to resist institutional control. By focusing so much on structural factors, it also overlooks the role of meaning and purpose in the lives of older people (Phillipson 1998). These latter issues have been central to a second form of critical thinking about later life, which has its origins in a more humanistic tradition.

Cultural and humanistic gerontology, sometimes referred to as moral economy because of its concerns with the ways in which social norms and reciprocal obligations influence the integration and social control of the elderly, has been particularly influential in the USA. Cole (1992), for example, argues that the study of aging had become too scientific by the beginning of the twentieth century, overlooking more existential and biographical concerns. This approach has been further developed by Moody (1993) who emphasizes the significance of meaning, interpretation and narrative in the construction of later life. Moody is critical of social gerontology for building on a form of rationalistic social science that is designed to predict and control human behaviour, arguing that this objectifies what is essentially a subjective experience. Instead, he calls for an emancipatory discourse and practice that goes further than simply offering negative critiques of current practice to suggest more positive ideas about human development. In essence, this means transcending conventional agist stereotypes about work and gender roles.

Recently, arguments have been made for bringing together the political economy model, with its emphasis on structured dependency, and the more humanistic and interpretative forms of theory. Phillipson (1998), for instance, has traced the ways in which the nature of aging changed in the latter half of the twentieth century, pointing to what he refers to as a 'crisis of identity' in older people. He argues that a critical gerontology must retain its concern with political economy but should also add a biographical and narrative perspective. From this comes a 'focus on the issue of empowerment, whether through the transformation of society (for example, through the redistribution of income and wealth), or through the development of new rituals and symbols to facilitate changes through the life course' (Phillipson 1998: 14). However, the incorporation of gender issues into this approach remains relatively underdeveloped and ethnicity has been virtually ignored.

The above views as to how theorizing later life should develop its critical edge and how ideas about culture and identity should be understood has also been challenged. Drawing on the postmodern notion of the 'cultural turn', Gilleard and Higgs (2000) argue for the significance of the consumer society in relation to later life. In the post-industrial era identity is no longer ascribed, stable or something that people are socialized into. Today identity is chosen and with the growth of consumerism it is made up of a large number of possible choices. This means that everyone, including older people, is involved in negotiating their identity and 'aging has become a much more reflexive project' (Gilleard and Higgs 2000: 25). Gilleard and Higgs claim that to understand aging we need to acknowledge that it occurs within an ever increasing number of cultural practices. Individuals are identified, and identify themselves, more through what they consume rather than by any intrinsic ascribable characteristics. They conclude that in these new times this 'applies as much to age and aging as it does to any other socialized attribute' (Gilleard and Higgs 2000: 25). However, they remain largely silent in terms of how gender and ethnicity might impinge on such a perspective. They also tend to overemphasize identity, subjectivity and culture to the neglect of material and other resources. The latter are arguably an important part of an individual's ability to participate fully in a consumer society and engage in allied identity creation. This is of particular significance to

35

older people, many of whom are victims of social exclusion on such grounds (Barnes et al. 2006).

A final approach, which has developed in response to the patholo-gizing of later life, concentrates on the positive aspects of growing older (Bytheway 1995; Biggs 1997). The emphasis here is on the ability of individuals to manage the aging process, remain active and resist the stereotypes of old age. Indeed, these are regarded as central to what is regarded as 'successful' aging. For instance, there is a chapter in a book by Bytheway (1995) called 'No more "elderly", no more age'. This relates to the 'mask of aging' theory, which suggests that there is really a youthful inner self trapped behind an aging exterior (Featherstone and Hepworth 1995). However, this arguably denies older people, especially older women, who are specifically required not to show their age, their greatest asset – their experience (Andrews 1999). Such an approach fails to shift the way in which older identities and bodies are constructed as subaltern to young identities and bodies. Rather, 'it perpetuates a cultural celebration of youthfulness and further stigma-tizes those elderly people who are outside the new frame of reference' (Irwin 1999: 695). It does not challenge the obsession with youth that dominates Western society but instead reinforces it. To this extent, despite the work of Torres (1999, 2003), it is also largely a culturally loaded approach. It is based on dominant assumptions about what constitutes contentment in later life, denying the diverse ethnic and cultural experiences of older people and the constellation of factors that contribute to their well-being.

As may be seen from the above discussion, theorizing about later life is increasingly developing. Attempts have been made to move on from the somewhat negative and deterministic views of the position of older people suggested by functionalist and political economy approaches. These have been countered by perspectives that are far more positive in orientation but which imply that aging can be overcome by buying into the consumer culture and remaining active. As Andrews has so suc-cinctly argued, 'this current tendency towards 'agelessness' is itself a form of ageism' (1999: 301). Further, as has been repeatedly pointed out, issues of gender and ethnicity remain properly to be addressed by mainstream gerontology theory. The next section will, therefore, consider insights to be gained from a feminist perspective.

Feminist perspectives on gender and aging

If gender and ethnicity have been relatively absent from theories about later life, it is also the case that older people have been largely hidden in both feminist theory and debates about ethnic relations. Whereas ideas about difference and diversity have been significant to feminist thinking for many years, the tendency has been to focus particularly on ethnicity and sexuality. Bradley (1996), who did discuss age in her book *Fractured Identities: Changing Patterns of Inequality*, sub-titled her chapter on this subject 'The Neglected Dimension of Stratification'. Women predominate in later life, their roles and relationships differ to those of men throughout the life course and their experiences of aging reflect this. It is strange then that feminists have largely failed to examine the interrelationship of sexism and ageism and how this affects women. Even when research has focused on older women, the tendency has been not to do this from a feminist perspective.

More recently, however, some feminists have been highlighting the neglect of gender issues in social gerontology. For example, in an early and highly influential text, Arber and Ginn (1991) asked why gender inequalities in later life had received such little attention? They examined the significance of gender differences among the elderly, particularly the key factors influencing independence and dependence. They also explored ageism and agist stereotypes, relating them to the gendered nature of power in society. Their analysis showed that older women are a significantly disadvantaged group in society.

Similarly, Bernard and Meade (1993) argued that older women experience the complex mixture of patriarchy and structural dis-advantage that younger women do but that age mediates and can profoundly change the nature of that experience. Their feminist agenda is to understand women's lives from a life course and multidisciplinary perspective. The former is significant since it recognizes the importance of individual history and the changing individual in a changing society. The latter is important because the multifaceted nature of that experience cannot be grasped using a particular disciplinary approach. A key argument is that 'it is the structures, policies and ideology of western capitalist society that are the major cause of women's relative social and economic powerlessness' (Bernard and Mead 1993: 1). Bernard and Meade conclude that to be an older woman is to be put in a contradictory position. Older women experience the impact of an agist and sexist society (and we might add other forms of diversity to this list) and suffer the effects of poverty and other forms of inequality. Yet, they may also live relatively satisfactory lives and are far from being passive victims. They also have much in common in terms of life experiences but many differences also exist. These influence the strengths they may bring to living through old age. This is something that is also supported by the research reported in this book.

There are, of course, many different kinds of feminist theory and it has been argued that each has something to offer us in thinking about later life (Browne 1998). However, the issue is not so much about imposing fixed theoretical frameworks on older women's experiences in the process of developing understandings and explanations of these. Rather, it is about how to go about theorizing these experiences, which does not necessarily mean taking existing theories as a starting point. Browne, for example, sees a feminist approach as focusing on women's lives in terms of the advantages and disadvantages that they derive from their gender, ethnic, class, age and other social positions (1998). She argues that it is about situating a gendered understanding of power as a collective, rather than an individual, phenomenon. She writes approvingly of MacKinnon's (1989) definition of feminist theory as being thinking that is 'critical of gender as a determinant of life chances' (Browne 1998: xxi). Browne also emphasizes that a feminist approach is about equality but that it is also about transforming society so that the latter recognizes that equality is an issue. Its aim is to eradicate ideologies and practices of domination and, thus, includes a commitment to anti-racism and challenging all forms of oppression. It would appear then that there is a synergy between social gerontology and feminism that could be taken further to good effect. While feminism recognizes the intrinsic value of women and their right to equality, gerontology is increasingly emphasizing the value of older people and their associated rights. It is time for feminists to suggest strongly that gerontology makes gender and diversity central to its concerns (Calasanti and Slevin 2001). This means more than just including gender as an interesting variable to be studied but involves incorporating it also as an analytical element in the generation of conceptual frameworks and understandings. Similarly, feminist theory on gender and difference more generally needs to become more sensitive to later life issues. Browne succinctly sums up the benefits to be gained from such an approach when she writes that:

> a feminist age analysis examines and critiques the underlying premises behind paradigms, policies, and programs that impact older women's lives, suggests a number of strategies to improve the lives of older women, and, ultimately, looks to a new epistemology of women and age for a more respectful vision for women – and men – in the later years. (Browne 1998: xxxv)

One example of a fruitful relationship between feminists and gerontologists is in thinking about the body. Although the body is an important signifier of age, it has not been a topic that has been given much attention in work on later life, except in the area of geriatrics. Here the focus has been on assessing the capability of an individual's body in order to assess that person's capacity to carry out independent tasks (Calasanti and Slevin 2001). Yet, as feminists have pointed out, the body is important for our self-identity and sense of self, particularly as we age and particularly for women. As Hockey and James (1993) indicate, the body has taken on great social significance in post-industrial society, with those that are young and lithe being the most acceptable. Anyone whose body does not visually conform to the current ideals may find that their social status and self-esteem is correspondingly reduced. Physical aging tends to be regarded in entirely negative ways, with various pills, potions, creams and surgical interventions available in order for youthfulness, supposedly, to be retained. Calasanti and Slevin (2001), for example, use the metaphor of 'war' in order to theorize what happens to the aging body. They argue that the dominant language in use suggests that we are constantly battling with our bodies as we are urged to 'fight', 'defy', 'mask' and 'eradicate' the signs of aging. Such fighting is, moreover, 'labour intensive'. Further, what they refer to as the 'politicization' of the body has led to increasing attempts by the state to regulate and manage it. For the elderly, as for others in the population, this means keeping active, eating healthily and trying to remain alert. The body serves as what Calasanti and Slevin refer to as a 'message board', which conveys age and gender-appropriate signs as to how well one is shaping up, as well as signals about ethnicity, class, ability, health and so on. For women, this emphasis on the body and on its appearance is central to how age-based bodily changes will be experienced and dealt with. For bodies have a materiality, which changes and on which cultural meanings are inscribed. They are not just symbolic or merely cultural sites (Hockey and James 2003). Thus, focusing on the interrelationship between sexism and ageism indicates that, despite the new rights and freedoms that women have won, new forms of oppression have arisen (Calasanti and Slevin 2001). Although men are also increasingly defined and judged by their body image, what Sontag (1978) dubbed the 'double standard of aging' nearly 30 years ago is still with us and ensures that the aging male is viewed less harshly than his female counterpart, as mentioned in the previous chapter. Further, a powerful media is increasingly able to reinforce this.

This discussion of the body is used as an example of what can be achieved theoretically when using a feminist-gendered lens. It is not just a case of adding women into existing gerontology theories, nor does it simply involve adapting feminist theory to take account of the elderly. Rather, it is a question of expanding and developing new concepts and views about what constitutes being old and the aging process. The body may be both a source of constraint and a resource in later life. It is also a vehicle through which older feminine and masculine identities are reproduced.

Ageing and ethnicities

As many commentators now acknowledge, there has been a lack of work that considers later life in relation to ethnicity (Butt and Moriart 2004; Nazroo et al. 2004). This is not so surprising given that, until recently as has already been seen, the ethnic minority populations in the UK have tended to have a younger demographic profile than the rest of the population, although this is changing. Where there is research on ethnic minority people in later life, this has tended to focus largely on health and social care. It has been suggested that they face a double or triple jeopardy as a consequence of their age, ethnic minority status and gender (Nazroo et al. 2004). However, there is an absence of theorizing exactly what this might mean.

One of the problems to be confronted when thinking about minority ethnic older people is that the theories and concepts that have been developed have almost exclusively focused on Western stereotypes of aging. Ultimately, this excludes, by definition, alternative under-standings and experiences of later life. In the subsequent chapters of this book we attempt to begin to remedy this situation. For example, in Chapter 6, on health and well-being, approaches based on uncritically applied Euro/American medicalized models are contested. Some of the concepts attached to what is meant by successful aging, such as autonomy, in/dependency, empowerment and agency cannot be effectively applied universally across culture, time and space. This is because they are linked to and rooted in liberalist accounts of the self and reason and the emergence of the cult of individualism. As Grim-shaw argues, 'the notion of the autonomy of the self and the autonomy of the individual desire is a liberalist individualist one' (Grimshaw 1986: 146). It is also one that has strongly influenced Western understanding of agency and (dis)empowerment and which has informed later life studies. Too often notions of liberal autonomy that polarize autonomy and dependence underpin agency and empower-ment. An effect of this is the association of power with independence and powerless with dependence. However, it is possible to be depen-dent without this posing a threat to autonomous or independent action and to be empowered and disempowered at the same time, as our research indicates.

It is for reasons such as these that we are attempting to develop what might be termed a 'post-gerontological' approach. The term is bor-rowed by analogy from Bracken and Thomas (2001) in their development of a post-psychiatry. Here different social and cultural contexts are central to unpicking psychiatry's largely Eurocentric construction of 'idioms of distress', while representing itself to be scientific and thus culturally neutral (Bracken and Petty 1998). Post-psychiatry takes the route of neither modernist psychiatry nor anti-psychiatry but looks for ways to affirm and learn from different cul-tural understandings. The parallels here with social gerontology in respect of its Westernism and Eurocentrism and assumptions of neu-trality are marked.

For us a post-gerontological stance would explore difference and the ways in which different cultures and systems of belief give meaning to stages and conditions of life and how these meanings might contribute to well-being in old age. It would explore the ways in which older people, in the case of our research older women from different backgrounds, empower themselves, as well as the ways in which they are disempowered. Our research, as detailed in the forthcoming pages, indicates that assumed structural disadvantages and constraints (health, housing, income, etc.) do not inevitably mean that women do not have the power to resist and transform their experiences of later life, although this may not preclude their need also for assistance. Our research indicates the potential of older women to be self-fulfilled through a variety of means. These include activities such as participation in voluntary and/or paid work, leisure pursuits, such as walking or dancing, religious activities, such as group prayers or bible-reading classes, attending lunch clubs and community centres, which provide opportunities for women to come together. The point is that these activities are not simply a reaction to the supposed disadvantages of later life, nor do they represent attempts to remain forever young. Rather, they represent the individual and collective creative capacity, purpose and agency of older women. The effects of material and structural conditions or access to resources do not negate this type of power.

One aspect of developing a post-gerontology approach involves deconstructing ideas about empowerment. Empowerment is a difficult term to define but finding an alternative one is equally problematic. Empowerment is not merely about giving services nor is it purely associated with 'doing' or agency. Feeling powerful or empowered has an ontological nature as well, a sense of self-worth that may indeed derive from cultural input and personal output, but which embraces a sense of value that enables a person to act and to receive. Foucault's (1979) theory has shown that power is differentiated and located. What is empowering or enabling for one person is not necessarily so for another and will vary according to life stages. We are exploring the ways in which our research participants are powerful and empowered using Jo Rowlands' (1998) paradigm of empowerment, which is constructed in the context of women and development in the Third World. Within development studies, empowerment discourse is frequently fashioned on the model of autonomy and its most conservative use may be limited to situations of self-help. The culture of autonomy does not favour many women, the old and the poor. Rowlands challenges the prioritization of an autonomous model of empowerment (based on the classical liberal model) and proposes an analysis that includes different models of power involving power-sharing. She suggests four kinds of power to which people might aspire: 'power over', relating to dominant hierarchical models (i.e. the traditional top-down model); 'power to'; 'power with' and 'power from within' (Rowlands 1998: 12). Rowlands argues that empowerment can be rooted in a person's own sense of identity, as well as shared with others. Our participants are mainly of two kinds; those who define their identity in relation to a collectivity and those who see themselves in terms of their individuality alone.

The appropriateness of Rowlands' model is evident in relation to the research presented in this book. For instance, the participants who came from the Commonwealth of Dominica some 40 years ago are empowered, but not in the white and generally masculine and con-sumerist ways of Western writing. They are empowered through their togetherness and collective activities (power with), as grandmothers (power over, power to, power with), through reciprocity and helping relationships (power to and power with) and through religion (power with and power from within). Many of these women are widows, with differing degrees of financial, health, transport and other difficulties. On Saturday nights they meet at the Association and there is dancing and music. They may celebrate Independence Day with a feast, which may include Caribbean music, dancing, storytelling and Caribbean food. They save small sums of money to afford the occasional outing. They smile, as one said, 'and look like the next sunny day'. They have a shared spirit of fight in them that keeps them going.

The accounts of the women in the research have also encouraged us to think of empowerment in other ways. First, there are different kinds of empowerment. Access to resources alone does not necessarily translate into empowerment but is also related to perceptions of their (that is the resources') value. As Kabeer notes:

> [a]ccess to new resources may open up new possibilities for women, but they are unlikely to seek to realise these possibilities in uniform ways. Instead, they will be influenced by the intersection of social relations and individual histories which form the vantage point from which they view these new possibilities. (1999: 460)

In this context culture is clearly highly important. Second, empowerment and disempowerment are relational concepts that have to be considered in the context of extent or degree. They are neither monolithic nor for all time articulating a process, rather than a definitive state that fluctuates and changes over time. Third, older women located in different cultural and geographical spaces can be simultaneously empowered and disempowered in different ways. Not only is this emphasis on contextuality important but people can be empowered in some areas of their lives and disempowered in others simultaneously. Finally, life course events, as well as current experiences, can influence both empowering and disempowering outcomes. Our women's different wartime and, for many, migratory experiences still affect their views of themselves and their lives today.

The post-gerontology described above underlies the general theoretical approach adopted in this book. Our aim is not to engage in abstract and cerebral thinking (this is not theory with a capital 'T'), nor is it merely to describe the 'findings' of the research, although clearly there are narratives and stories to be told. Rather, we are engaged in what Layder (1998) calls 'adaptive' or Mouzelis (1991) 'middle-range' theory, where ideas and concepts are linked together as they emerge from empirical research. In adopting this style of working, we want to develop news ways of thinking about and understanding the subject matter of each chapter. The aim is to begin to think about how we might generate more sensitive and less culturally specific meanings. This is done with a view to rendering visible ethnic and cultural experiences of later life, which have often been hidden from view.

Researching gender, ethnicity and later life: some methodological issues

A number of methodological issues arose as a result of conducting this research. The first was the issue of selecting a group of participants within the three ethnic groups named on the proposal: African-Caribbean, Asian and white able-bodied women. The recruitment of ethnic minorities to research is beginning to generate an interesting literature (Cook et al. 2004; Holland 2005; Sin 2005). Many of our Asian and African-Caribbean participants were recruited through community centres. This is not always a good approach to adopt since it means going through gatekeepers and might be seen as lazy, although in our case it was a way of dealing with the fact that both our main researchers were white and we needed to work with sensitivity. However, an unforeseen issue that arose was that one group of African-Caribbean elders claimed that they were being over-researched. They were angry at being asked the same questions again and again, with no obvious outcomes or change in their circumstances. Similarly, at a Bangladeshi centre there were four research projects already in a queue waiting for the opportunity to conduct interviews. Research burn-out is a real issue here and is likely to become more serious the more researching ethnic minority elders moves higher up the research agenda. Moreover, it was a problem encountered by other projects on the Growing Older Programme (Scharf 2005).

In contrast, however, the Polish women, together with a group of white inner-city women living in sheltered housing, expressed anger at never being asked for their opinion and felt that they were constantly being overlooked. The latter reported that stones were regularly thrown at their windows and that they saw themselves as being under siege. Such white inner city women are not in demand as research subjects and do not, in the main, attract research funding, although the recent work by Scharf et al. (2005) is one exception to this. There is a need, therefore, to ensure that we are as inclusive as possible when researching later life. This is likely to become increasingly difficult as the range of cultures represented within the UK enlarges.

At the outset of the research we decided to deconstruct the ethnic categories described in the proposal in order to show difference. For instance, not all South Asian people are Muslims or Indian or Pakistani. Neither is 'white' a homogeneous group. The black Caribbean women came from different Caribbean islands but they did not necessarily have a shared identity. The racism that our black Caribbean participants have experienced in Britain makes them feel that they are, as one put it, 'all in the same boat'. However, there were clear differences between island cultures that could still be distinguished, even 40 years after migration. Further, many older women did not like the term 'African-Caribbean', saying that they did not see themselves as 'African'. So this is an ascribed category for many of them, who preferred to be called West Indian or Caribbean. There is an issue, however, in relation to these differences within differences and minorities within minorities, about how far researchers can go in dealing with them. How far is it possible to go in deconstructing difference, given constraints of time and budget, and how far is it possible to make a reasoned decision? There are many differences within minority ethnic groups in our research location. Within the Pakistani Muslim community, for example, there are Pathans who speak Pushtu, Attocks and Mirpuris and so on. Within the Indian community, there are Gujaratis who speak a different language from the Punjabis. Members of the Indian community may also be Hindus, Muslims or Sikhs. These different identities mean that our respondents had disparate, as well as shared, views on aging and the meaning of later life, even within ethnic groupings. It is difficult to ensure that these are fully represented within the confines of one research project. It would have been impossible also to ask about sexuality, although sexual orientation is another largely hidden aspect in research on later life.

The issue of difference also raises problems at the analysis stage of research. The more difference is emphasized, the more complex the data that is generated, and this makes difficulties for analysis. It is not easy to disentangle overlapping issues and to make sense of which are the most significant in influencing a person's views and experiences. One issue which arose, particularly in the research, relates to religion because it was not a form of difference that we had initially expected to research. However, as Chapter 6 makes clear, faith or spirituality was important for most of our participants, even those who are white. Yet, it is not always clear how religion and ethnicity may be separated, as the discussion in the above paragraph indicates. Further, given the current public focus on the Muslim religion, and the Islamophobia that has ensued, it is going to be necessary to pay much more attention to religion in later life research in the future, given that it has not been given much consideration up until now (Afshar et al. 2005a, b).

Other methodological matters were also raised during the course of the research. Whereas the Polish women wanted to tell their stories, which they felt were not well known outside of their community, the Pakistani women, we were told, often got paid for interviews. This was not possible as such payments had not been included in the research budget. It raises questions about bargaining and 'trade-offs'. Two interim reports and a summary of the final report were circulated, in order to keep participants informed and allow for feedback. When the fieldwork was completed, all participants were invited to a meeting at the University of York, with transport provided, to thank them for their help, present some preliminary findings and hear their views. One hundred and forty people attended and, after a meeting and lunch, they were taken for an outing in the city. This was part of the trade-off we had offered them. Though not without its hiccups, this day proved to be a great success. In general, however, there needs to be more discussion concerning trade-offs with participants in research work.

A final methodological issue for discussion involves the use of interpreters for some of the interviews and there are many ways in which this was not ideal. Financial constraints limited the number of interpreters who could be employed. Sometimes volunteers were used, raising issues about the exploitation of those who offered their services. Sometimes it was necessary to interview participants in their second language, thereby putting pressure on the interviewee. Further, there can be a discrepancy between the length of an interview and the amount of information gained, since it may take longer to obtain the same level of response when having to translate, which is tiring for all concerned. Interviews that ended at an average length of time for the project overall may not yield a similar amount of transcript. Moreover, some interpreters talked about the interviewee in the third person and this meant that we did not get access to direct quotes. In any case, it is not possible to obtain direct quotes as such, when the quote is translated into another language and language plays a pivotal role in the construction of meaning (Jentsch 1998; Temple and Edwards 2002). Temple, for example, who has a particular interest in using interpreters and translators in cross-language research, has highlighted the sensitivities involved when selecting particular words for a translation (1997). This is because words are used to describe experience and may do so in a culturally particular way, thereby defining some people as 'outsiders'. She notes that '[W]hen different languages are used there is an obvious mechanism for excluding someone' (Temple 1997: 611). Twyman et al. (1999) have also suggested the necessity to explore the positionality of 'self' and 'other' in relation to using interpreters and translation. They write, '[i]n essence, this requires a shift from researcher as observer to researcher as observed, and with this an emergence of self-reflexive and context laden fieldwork' (Twyman et al. 1999: 323). This highlights the importance of taking notes and keeping diaries during the fieldwork and using them as part of the analysis.

Issues to do with power also arose when it was necessary to work with male interpreters or through interpreters who knew the interviewees or those who were acting as volunteers. These people may have their own particular agendas, which may not be apparent to those from outside the community, and they may use the interview as an opportunity for ventriloquism. One possibility for combating any likely interpreter bias was to have the whole interview transcribed by a separate translator. However, there are ethical (and financial) issues in relation to this and also those of access. It would not be ethical to translate the entire interview, without the permission of both inter-viewee and interpreter, and there can be no linguistically absolute translation. In addition, interviewer and interpreter would need to be aware of the intent to translate the whole interview from the outset.

Another factor in thinking about power relations and interpreting is that where the interpreter and the interviewee share a language, this may well give them a sense of private space into which the actual researcher may not step and that this may be reassuring to the inter-viewee. But the power relations between the interpreter and the interviewee are not always obvious and neither are those between the researcher and the interpreter. Jentsch (1998), for example, refers to a situation where she felt under pressure from the evaluation of her performance by a male interpreter, who had interpreted for a previous interviewer with the same interviewee. In our research a male inter-preter, who was also a community leader, was used at a Gujarati Hindu Centre, where none of the women spoke any English. The community leader offered to translate our interview topic guide into Gujarati and to give the questions to the women in the senior citizens' group to answer. The community leader then interpreted the answers for the researcher. Although unconventional, this was not a wasted process. Despite the obvious power relationship between the interpreter and the respondents, the answers provided did offer important cultural insights into the lives of these older Indian women and into the breakdown of the joint family situation. Further, the answers acted as a means of gaining access for interviews in the homes of three Gujarati women, two of whom lived alone and one of whom lived in the joint family situation but who wanted to live on her own. The translated topic guide, together with the resulting interviews, overturned some of the stereotypes about older Indian women and the joint family, thereby indicating the benefits that may accrue from sometimes moving away from a straightforward methodological agenda.

Conclusion

This chapter has sought to explore some of the general debates around the use of theory in studying later life. It has looked at some of the issues that arise from employing a feminist perspective and gendered lens and has argued for a middle-range approach in generating theoretical understandings and meanings. The chapter has raised questions about theoretical work in relation to aging, gender and ethnicity and has suggested that what has been termed as a 'post-gerontology' approach might help to make visible hidden cultural assumptions and stereotypes in ideas and concepts. It discussed how new ways of thinking about (dis)empowerment have arisen from our theoretical engagement with our empirical material.

The final part of the chapter considered some of the methodological issues that have arisen from doing cross-cultural research with older minority ethnic women in the UK. While more questions than answers have emerged, we suggest that these and other matters require airing, particularly since the UK is becoming an even more diverse multicultural society than ever.

We offer these insights as a framework for the book. However, it is the lives, experiences and voices of our older women participants that are of major concern. These are now highlighted in the pages that follow.

Identities and life course events

Introduction

Identity has become an important concept in recent decades because it links individuals to the society in which they live. One's identity is about belonging and is marked by both similarity and difference. It relates both to what people have in common with one another and what differentiates them (Woodward 2003). As is increasingly acknowledged, each individual incorporates a whole range of identities, which are part of everyday life. These identities are experienced and constructed out of a myriad of daily interactions with others, involving the interchange and negotiation of how one sees oneself with how we believe others see us. Further, taking on an identity often means more than simply acting out a role. We tend to have considerable amounts of personal, and often collective, investment in the identities we adopt (Woodward 2003). This means that having some understanding of who we are is crucial to notions of self and contributes to our sense of worth and well-being.

As discussed in the previous chapter, commentators on later life have tended to portray it either as an inevitable stage when roles and faculties are lost, resulting in disengagement with society, or as a period when older people should be actively working to age 'successfully'. In the former, identity is passively restricted. In the latter, the emphasis is on agency and choice. However, some older people have more scope for negotiating their identities than others, since economic, material and physical constraints can limit options. Further, an older person's sense of who they are may be particularly influenced by life course events. Specific personal circumstances and individual biographies, together with particular historical and political occurrences, may all contribute to how they view themselves (Bradley 1996).

This chapter examines some of the main issues relating to identity and the life course, with reference to later life, as discussed by women from a range of ethnic groups. It begins by looking at some ethnic differences in how women perceived age and the notion of being 'old'. It then considers some of the complexities in how older women define themselves in terms of ethnicity and nationality. The next section looks at the women's experiences of war and other conflicts, as well as focusing on the migratory process and its consequences. This is followed by a discussion of racism, mainly through the experiences of first generation African-Caribbean women. The significance of employment and retirement is then explored. Finally, the conclusion indicates that for the migrant women, the migratory process itself is particularly significant. In addition to being highly stressful and disruptive, racism also served to construct them as 'different' and as minority ethnic groups. The significance of these relatively early experiences remain with them today. However, they still have a clear sense of their own hyphenated identities.

Gender, ethnicity and age

The often complex life courses of our participants made it impossible to think of them as having a single identity. The multiplicity, fluidity, contextualized and contested qualities of identities that studies of gender have highlighted have undermined any notion of a single, all-embracing, primary identity to which all others must be subordinated (Eley and Suny 1996). Women often have more fluid identities than men. They are named after their fathers and, subsequently, their husbands, and are known as the mothers of their children. In addition to the nomenclature, life processes mark women physically and psychologically (Hockey and James 2003). After giving birth, women experience the physical and emotional changes that accompany the move from being an individual to being recognized as someone's mother. The physical alterations and the developments that mark a woman's body have hormonal, as well as psychological changes, that affect all women, whether or not they are mothers.

In terms of identity, there were differences in how the women in this study felt in different phases of their lives in relation to aging. Pakistani and Bangladeshi women, for instance, reported identifying as 'old' at an earlier age than other participants, suggesting that they saw themselves in this way at 50 or even 40 years old. These perceptions were related to the transitions associated with rites of passage, such as marriage, becoming a grandparent or bereavement, events marking a stage in a woman's advance through life. A Pakistani woman, who was widowed when her children were small, stated that she had started to feel old after her husband died. Another indicated that, since she got married at 13 and was a grandmother at 35 years of age, it was at that point that she felt old. Some of the African-Caribbean respondents stated that the responsibilities they had felt at an early age meant that they also felt old when they were young. However, identifying as old had waned as these responsibilities themselves decreased. One participant, for example, who had given birth to four children in four years, reported that, paradoxically, she regarded herself as younger now that she was over 60 than she had done while bringing up her children. This indicates that perceptions of self in relation to age do not necessarily have to follow a linear progression.

All this may be contrasted to women from India and Poland, for example, who said that they would not regard themselves as being old until they were virtually incapacitated. As one Indian woman put it: 'a person is old when the body is not working'. Another said that she considered a woman to be old: 'when she can't do anything in the house. As long as you are moving around, you are alright'. A similar view was expressed by a Polish respondent, who thought that a woman was old when: 'she has illness and nobody understands this'. She also linked old age to lack of control, which was brought about by ill-health, such as Alzheimer's disease:

> If you lose control about yourself and your life and you can't do any other and you rely on the other people, which is very hard. You have not your own voice, you know. Your voice is nothing. Yes. They do instead of you. They tell you.

Further, the majority of all first generation migrant women felt that they were not treated any differently in later life than they had been in their earlier years. They pointed out that there is respect for elders in their cultures, although a small number, mainly from the Pakistani and Indian communities, spoke of how this was beginning to break down due to Western cultural influences and the erosion of joint family living arrangements. An Indian respondent told us that her culture's emphasis on respect for the elderly contributed to older people's quality of life. Another indicated:

> we do have to respect our elders. We have to respect those older. It is our duty. That's how we've been brought up. Maybe it will be different when our children grow up.

It was mainly the white non-migrant women who brought up the issue of having their identity eroded, of being made to feel invisible and of being ignored or dismissed because of their perceived age. In fact, a number of white working class respondents indicated that as older women they did not feel that they got enough respect, with one commenting that she was treated:

> As though you're not there. You don't belong. I mean, I was always brought up to respect older people. We don't get enough respect. They think you're simple if you're getting old but they don't understand some of us have got better brains than what they have.

This view was supported by other white working class women, two of whom indicated that:

> we don't matter now, we older people, we don't matter now.

> A lot of people, a lot of our age group feel the same. We're just being pushed to the back and others are being brought forward to take over, That's it in a nutshell.

The white middle-class women also reported feeling the same way. One said:

> I think going into shops and you are not a nonentity but you are not looked at anymore. Oh dear! I don't know. I feel that when someone is kind to you and talks to you, it's the exception rather than the rule, you know.

Another woman reported having similar shopping experiences:

> And I'm sure its something to do with they think you are a bit dithery, because of your age you see.

However, there was evidence of resistance to aegist stereotypes. Some of the white women also reported that being older enabled them to say more outrageous and outspoken things because they no longer cared about their image or what people were thinking about them. Supportive women friends and networks also provided a social resource for entering public spaces collectively and asserting a collective older identity, by being seen and acting together.

Thus, ethnic and cultural differences influence the way in which older women see themselves in terms of age and how they believe others perceive them. For some, there appears to be no boundary to be crossed into 'old age', certainly while they are able to 'keep going'. For others, boundaries do exist, which relate both to personal history and to cultural practice. Further, what is meant by 'old', how it is experienced and identified with mean different things in different contexts. While for many of our white British-born women their age becomes, what Wilson (2000) has referred to as a distancing mechanism, signifying their difference and constructing them as 'other', many of the migrant women consider it to be a resource that ties them to community bonds. For such women, aging becomes an achievement, rather than a negative ascription.

Ethnicity, nationality and identification

As previously described, we sought to work with three groups: African-Caribbean, Asian and white women. However, researchers face many problems in defining 'ethnicity' (Fine et al. 1997; Brown et al. 1999; Bulmer and Solomos 2004). It has been argued that 'black' and 'white' are no longer useful categories for understanding the situation of minority ethnic groups in Britain (Modood et al., 1997). In the past, there has also been a tendency to 'over-racialize' the categories of African-Caribbean and Asian and de-racialize groups, such as the Irish and Eastern Europeans rendering them invisible under the cloak of 'whiteness', although political debate over the European Union (EU) accession states makes this less likely for current Eastern European migrants these days (Mac an Ghaill 1999). As discussed in Chapter 3, there are differences not only within African-Caribbean and Asian people, but also within white groups (Bulmer and Solomos 2004), none of which should be glossed over.

With the increase of Islamophobia following the 9/11 attacks in the USA and the 7/7 bombings and repeat attempts in London, the problems of defining ethnicity have arguably moved from the realm of the academic to that of politics. There have been demands, for example, by Hazel Blears, a former Minister of Multiculturalism, that minority ethnic groups should take on a more specifically British ethnic identity. The suggestion is that people should be able to lead different, but not separate lives. So, in her series of meetings with Muslims during the summer of 2005, one question that the Minister reportedly planned to ask was:

> would they rather be termed 'British-Asian' or Indian-British rather than simply Muslim or Asian? (*The Times* 2005)

However, none of our Asian respondents saw themselves as being 'simply' Muslim or Asian in this way. Such a nomenclature would have created for them merely an ascribed identity, one that hid, rather than explained, much about how they defined themselves (Afshar et al. 2005a). Although 'Asian' people may be largely perceived from the outside to be homogenous within these communities, as described in Chapter 2, there are differences of language and religion (Bradford Health Authority 2001). There are also many differences even within the Pakistani Muslim communities. For instance, the Pathans who speak Pushtu come from a different part of Pakistan to the Attocks, who have distinct and different cultural norms and practices from the Mirpuris and so on. Similarly, the black Caribbean women in our sample came from different Caribbean Islands. The racism that the black Caribbean participants experienced in the UK has given them a sense of unity but has not necessarily made them feel that they have shared identities. The ascribed categories 'black' or African did not suit many of the women, who preferred to be recognized by their birthplace rather than by the colour of their skin. African-Caribbean people may be put together as a single otherised group by some observers and sometimes by members of the younger British-born generation in the UK. However, the older generation remembers that they were born as Barbadians, Jamaicans, and so on. It is younger generations who may be more likely to have formed a common ethnic identity. Thus, while an 'ethnic group' such as the African-Caribbean 'may be defined as one that shares a common past or history, it is important to remember that the past has different meanings for different age groups' (Blakemore and Boneham 1994: 57).

The women to whom we talked did not necessarily define themselves in terms of their nationality or ethnicity (Schmidt 2002). But the self-ascribed identities that they chose to construct, within the constraints of their social/political/personal circumstances, were sometimes anchored in their faith, leading to definitions that crossed traditional divides, both personally and politically (Vermeulen and Govers 1994; Ghorashi 2003). They were often constructed through their lived experiences and through encounters with the host society and its agencies. For the first generation of migrants, particularly when among their kin group, there is little need to define what is meant by identity, since there are clear points of reference, particular places, people and stories that can be repeated in relation to this (Afshar 1989a). They know where they came from, why they came and who they were before the migration (Afshar 1994). They define themselves in terms of the kin groups that they left behind, their social position and the locality in which they had grown up.

Our participants described their own ethnicities in terms of a range of allegiances and experiences. Their sense of who they are is inter-woven with religious, national, cultural and linguistic pasts and histories that, combined with their ethnic origins, create their own sense of self. Some were clear about a particular identity, defining themselves in terms of the country or the province that was their birth place. Some of our respondents simply said that they were Indian, while others saw themselves as Gujaratis. Some wished to be more specific, making distinctions between being 'Pakistanis' and 'Northern Pakistanis'. Others again defined themselves in terms of their faith, particularly the Muslims. However, most of the women who had migrated to the UK needed a wider categorization. The move from birthplace to where they live now, sometimes passing through a different continent on the way, had given many of our participants a fluid and hyphenated sense of identity. Asked to define her ethnicity, one woman said: 'I'm a black person ... we came from Africa ... I am black West Indian'. Yet, remembering where they came from did not make the women definitively who they were. They also saw themselves as British. So this participant also thought of herself as British Jamaican, as did a number of other women from this island background.

Other women also emphasized their Britishness by referring to themselves as 'British Muslims'. However, this was sometimes qualified, as when a Pakistani woman told us that after 38 years in Britain, she felt 'more British than anything else' and that she no longer felt any sense of belonging when she visited her family in Pakistan. Another woman, who was originally from Kenya, said that she was a 'British Muslim'; she had lived in the UK for 34 years. A further respondent, who is 64, said via an interpreter:

> I am a British Muslim. But because I belong to Pakistan, I am Pakistani as well, I still have my family there and I still go back.

A Polish woman responded that she was: 'well both Polish and British'.

These women's self-identities do not necessarily accord with ascribed identities, such as those of 'immigrant', 'Muslim' or 'Irish,' with which they are faced. Such ascriptions have internal and external impacts on the women and their kin group and help to reproduce a 'structure, which is manifesting new patterns of social marginalisation', especially for Muslim women or those who are thought to be Muslim (Irwin 1999: 712).

For some women also, the past has been so painful that they have no wish to return to their country of origin and often have no place or relatives to return to. These women emphasized their British identity because they have no alternative. As one Polish woman said, there was no return for her:

> Because we could not go back to Poland because Poland was occupied first by the Germans and the other side by the Russians, but when the Germans were defeated in 1945, so the Russians occupied the whole [of] Poland for 50 years. Just the last 10 years Poland is free ... that's why we are in England because our Poland was occupied by Russia. But when the war started the Russians occupied us ...

Although she sees herself as 'both Polish and British', her Poland no longer exists.

> I have nobody. I not even write a letter because I have nobody. Nobody. That place where I used to live before is under Belorussia now. Even if I want to go and see there's nothing. I can't. I have nobody there. I even not write letters because I have nobody there. Now I have British authorisation. I have British passport.

For this respondent, as for others from Poland, the latter was no longer a piece of land and a geographical entity. Rather, it was a social gathering of like-minded people, with a shared history, at the Polish club. It was a Poland that could only be found in England:

> after church [we go to] club just next door. Having a cup of coffee and cake and waiting until two o'clock for our bus. There are seven of us travelling. So we are like a little piece of Poland when we come here. So thank God I am British!

Nevertheless, some of our respondents were keen to transmit the history of their lives and migration to their descendants. Many talked about their past with longing and affection, and one participant had begun writing about it for her descendants, which was not always as easy task. The Polish participants were particularly keen on retaining their language. As one pointed out, one of the pleasures in her life was to come to the community centre where she could talk her 'head off in Polish'. For them, it was important to transfer that identity to their children and grandchildren by holding onto their language.

In contrast, most of the non-migrant white British women did not respond to questions about ethnicity and nationality in such complex or detailed terms. Most replied that they were white English or white British and could see no reason why there should be further discussion about this. It was just how they were, how they saw themselves and how they expected others to see them. The white inner-city women saw themselves as straightforwardly English and for them it was, as one woman put it, 'as plain as that'. However, they also expressed concern about what they perceived to be an erosion of their Englishness. This was articulated not only in terms of feeling threatened by minority ethnic people but also by the Welsh, the Scots and the EU. One woman said she thought that, 'English people have been pushed under the carpet. This is what I feel anyway, very strongly'. Another stated that, 'All our cultures are being swept away'. The view was expressed that, 'While Scotland has got Scotland and Wales have got Wales ... English is just being pushed to the back'. There were further objections to the idea that they were being made to think of themselves as Europeans, with views that the EU had 'taken over', that 'we are the ones that are the underdogs' and 'we're all individual nations ... and they don't give a damn about us ...' being expressed. These women also objected to the fact that they did not feel free to express their views because if they tried to say anything they were accused of being racist. They lived in an area where they often had stones thrown at their windows and perceived themselves to be somewhat under siege. They were discontented and prey to neo-fascist propaganda that came through their letter boxes. They felt that they had to defend their identity as being English at all costs because, as one contributor put it, 'we feel as though we've lost our country'.

Wartime experiences and the migration legacy

All our participants were of an age to have experienced some of the 20th century wars and upheavals, and their lives had been marked by these. Wartime memories and experiences were very influential in the lives of the Polish and African-Caribbean women and had an important impact on the lives of many of the white non-migrant British women. These early biographical experiences not only had lasting consequences for how women saw themselves, but they also had implications and repercussions for subsequent life course events, which in themselves had implications for the women's identity now.

For instance, most of the African-Caribbean women had come to the UK during the 'migration boom' of the 1940s and 1950s, which caused considerable social upheaval. The out-migration of the young ablebodied at that time caused 'acute distress' both to older people and the children left behind (Lowenthal 1972: 220). Many of these migrants, who are now growing old themselves, have had to try to come to terms with the impact of their departure and arrival in a new land (Blakemore and Boneham 1994). We were told that, 'I don't think nobody came into this country and had life easy, no' and

> when I came here the work I used to do at home and what the job I started doing, I would never have done it at home. But for the benefit of my children, I decided to do the job I did [working in a factory which bottled fizzy drinks].

Some of our respondents came to this country without any kin support group. Some had left after invasions, occupations or expulsions. Some were second-time migrants of Indian origin, leaving Uganda after military dictator Idi Amin announced his plans to expel them. Others were Poles, who had been moved to camps in Russia and from there to camps in the UK. Many had not expected to end up in the UK. As one Ugandan-Asian woman put it:

> When we were in Africa we never even thought or dreamt that we would leave Africa one day. You see we were there born there.

She went on:

> All the, the, the hard work of our lifetime, all whatever we, we made, our homes everything, our properties, everything we just left the house full of all our lifetime earning and we just left with only few clothes and we left. I used to cry so much ... we came and we went straight into the camp. You left your wonderful home and you came to stay in a camp. It was such a nightmare and my husband used to watch me cry all the time ...

Migration had been hard for all who had experienced it and we heard tragic stories about terrible journeys across countries or continents and harrowing memories of loss and hardship. The histories that led to second-time migrations and the hardships that had been endured were almost unimaginable. The Polish participants remembered the horrors of their lives during the Second World War. Wartime experiences came up, particularly in the interviews with both Polish white non-migrant British women, who talked about their memories, feelings, then and now, and the impact of these on their sense of self. For the Polish participants, for instance, war meant extreme hardship, including deportation as teenagers to become forced labour in Germany or the USSR, loss of their families and a changed geography of their homeland, as they knew it. A 79-year-old Polish woman told her story to Myfanwy Franks:

> In September the war start. 19th of September. But when the war started the Russia occupy us. So I only [lived] with my mother. And we were deported to Siberia working in the forest .... I was 18 ... Nine months is snow in Siberia. My mother died 7 May. It was still with snow. And they have to dig in the snow. Dig in the ground because, you know, it was frozen and bury without coffin like a dog. My mother died after three months because all old people and all children die because hungry and cold. We (were) very hungry, very short of food. Terrible. Terrible. And for two years it was like that in 1944 ... So when the war was finished Germany have to go out from Poland but Russia hold the whole country.

So we were out already. Out of our country ... Many had been in Russia.
Many had been in Germany. Many had been murdered in concentration
camp ... Winston Churchill and Roosevelt and Stalin at the meeting
organised the army. So the Stalin let us out and England took us over ...
The Polish men were in the Polish army but under British rule completely and were in British uniform. We women, young and single,
volunteered. So, I go voluntary because I was single then only twenty.
Not married yet. No family ... And when I joined the army we have to
have medical examination. You know how much I weigh? 4 stone and 6
pounds.

Another Polish woman could remember the exact date of her
deportation:

It was my birthday and it's significant to me because just on that day all
the families were taken to Russia ... It was 10th February 1940 ...
Germans came over from West and they [Russians] came from East and
they met on river there. They divided Poland between themselves and we
were living on the eastern part of Poland and in 1940 first deportations to
Russia was 10 February 1940 ... So we were taken from Poland by a
goods train. A lot of people in one compartment, you know, and there's
no toilet or anything like that. We have to cut a hole in the floor to do
our business. Yes, there was no food or anything like that. No hot water
during the day. They usually knocked and opened the doors and gave us
some hot water or sometimes we have to get out and gather the snow. It
was winter, very hard winter then, very, very hard winter – frost and a lot
of snow. So we were gathering snow and making water to drink. Of
course, they allowed us to take some food, you know. We didn't have
much. Couldn't get much because there was a limited time to pack things
... We travelled from 10 February until Easter ... We travelled there in
that goods train. It's not Siberia actually. Tundra or something like that,
Archangelsk. Do you know where Archangelsk is? [Near the White Sea
on the border of Siberia]. Yes we were a bit south of those forests ...
where we stayed about two years working. Felling trees, you know,
cutting. Doing in the forest whatever it was there to do. The hardest work
was to fell trees you know ... It was 1942, August, when I left Russia and
my father left Russia then. He joined the army. My husband, he wasn't
my husband then. A lot of people, 100,000 soldiers, plus families and we
went to Persia – it is Iran, Iran – and we stayed there for a while and then
families. I have met my father there and my mother and the rest of the
family. We were in tents on the beach on the Caspian Sea. We came

through Caspian Sea onto Iran on a beach and then from there we were taken by British to all sorts of places. India, South Africa and those families stayed there [during the rest of] the war and my father went with the army to Italy and he was fighting at Monte Cassino … Anyhow, when the war ended May 18 1945, so the army stayed a while in Italy having a rest and then came over to England. And some of course families from India or Africa joined fathers who were soldiers and came over here. Some people went to Poland. Not many. Of course British government wanted us to go home. Yes, they were actually persuading us, you know. Usually a gentleman came. He talked to us and wanted as many as possible to go home. Some of the people went and they landed back in Siberia.

This was one of the many stories of suffering and hardship that the Polish women carry about the war with its lasting effects. Most of them could not speak English when they arrived. Their schooling had been interrupted and for some it was never resumed. This meant that they were not able to obtain qualifications, with resulting consequences for employment, income and life chances. Most of the Polish women in this study worked in the textile industry. Those women who were old enough to work on their arrival in the UK reported how they were not initially able to choose employment for themselves but were told what to do. This meant that at first they did the jobs that nobody else wanted. As one woman explained:

Yes, for some time we've got the identity cards and we couldn't move without notifying police we are moving there. We supposed to work two years in mill to which they had taken us.

Another described how frightened she was when she first went to work at burling (picking knots out of material) and mending:

So I was given a table and tools and pieces and there was a lady who was teaching us to do it. It was very, very difficult because we didn't understand what she was talking. I had never been in a factory. I had *never* seen a piece of seventy yards long and that wide [extends hands], which were usually sixty inches wide. So it was everything very, very new to me.

These women also described how the British authorities seemed neither to be prepared for the arrival of the Polish migrants nor to have any plans to teach the newcomers what to expect of the UK – complaints made also by the African-Caribbean women. They felt that 'we were not very welcome, no'.

> And because of that, we suffered a lot. We had a really hardship here because the first winter was very cold. We had been very poorly dressed because it was the war, so we didn't have any clothes and there was no means of getting anything and then nobody bothered with us here ... They didn't even bother to put a bed sheet ... There was no hot water to have a bath or proper wash.

The Polish women spoke of how their wartime and migratory experiences had affected them greatly. Although not dwelling on these experiences now, they mostly remember everything that happened to them and think about them 'all the time'.

Those older women who had grown up in India or Pakistan would have lived through the time of India's independence (1947) and the momentous and terrible events following the partition of India and Pakistan. These many changes 'are woven into the past of older Asian people now living in Britain' (Blakemore and Boneham 1994: 77). Yet, in contrast to the Polish women's voluble statements about the war, Indian and Pakistani participants did not speak about the violence in their countries in the interviews. It seems that sometimes memories are too painful to be revisited lightly and, particularly in a subcontinent as large as India, momentous events may have passed unnoticed. When one Indian respondent was asked why she had not mentioned Partition, she replied that she did not do so because it had had very little effect upon her.

Although these women spoke about being 'surprised' and 'shocked' when they arrived in the UK because it was 'an alien land' and most of them did not speak English, they generally said that they were pleased to be here because it meant being with their husbands, children and family. A second-time migrant, a Gujarati, who came to the UK from Uganda, could remember the exact date of her arrival. 'I've been here since 1947 28th February'. But for her migration was a happy experience. She said: 'I like I came to this country and everybody's happy'. She said that she could even cope with the hardest thing, which was the cold:

> It doesn't bother me because I'm young and my husband was here. You know, Gujarati, when they came from East Africa, they find it very different but I didn't mind.

The majority of Pakistani and Bangladeshi women lacked education and due to poor or non-existent English had never worked outside the home. Instead, they had worked in the household and had sometimes contributed to family-run businesses. Those who did work had done so mainly in mills and textile factories. Many of these older women migrants, despite claiming to be content in the UK, continue to look back with longing at their previous homelands, doing so through the tinted glasses of memory. One woman, who had lived in England for 36 years, told us through an interpreter:

> What she's saying that, you know, for her the good life was in India because she says she didn't have to worry about anything. Paying this, pay that bill and they were living happily, no worries, eating and sleeping without any worry. But since they have come to this country, all the worries have started and the biggest problem is money. She said, you know, we do want to go out, we do want to enjoy our lives after all this hard work, but we can't afford it with this amount of money.

Similarly, the African-Caribbean women had clear and fond memories of their homelands. Reminiscing about where she came from, one respondent told Myfanwy Franks:

> Well I would describe it as a friendly place, you know. Easy life. We haven't got a lot but we were always happy. Even though we were a big family I originally come from, which is like six brothers and six sisters, we were all fed and looked after. We didn't have a lot of money but we had more than most people because what we had we had to work together to do it. It was somebody had to go to the garden to get vegetables provision. We had cattle which somebody had to feed. Everybody had their job individual. Everybody had their job and you know what's expected of you as you [get] bigger. When crop was due. All the year round there's something that's ready for cultivating. It could be oranges. It could be cocoa beans, coffee beans, vanilla, ginger, you know. We sell bananas. We take bananas to the market to sell. And we would get a cow ready and we had pigs and everything, you know, and we would kill one for Christmas and we'd smoke it, that's what we used to do ... and we were all very happy. If my dad could afford a bottle of wine he would get a bottle of wine and everybody would have a sip, you know. He would give each and every one of us a sip.

Another African-Caribbean woman also told us about her early life:

I enjoyed life growing up. I had a real happy life growing up, you know. We used to go all around on the bikes, you know. From St Patrick's Day on, the weather was getting good and we'd go, every Sunday every Saturday, and we'd finish walking our bikes, you know, all around everywhere. We'd a right enjoyable life and then summer holidays come and we used to go on holiday, usually down the country about thirteen/ fourteen miles. We used to go down there for six weeks of our holidays, you know. We enjoyed life in every way, you know. And even at home we'd a right happy family life, you know.

Nonetheless, a Dominican contributor talked about the Caribbean men who gave their lives as servicemen fighting for the UK, and the women who became nurses to care for the wounded. She felt disgust at how their contribution is seldom remembered. This is also the case in terms of the many Polish combatants who gave their lives, as well as those from the Indian subcontinent.

The experiences, deprivations and sacrifices of white people living in the UK at the time of the Second World War are well recorded (Braybon and Summerfield, 1986; Summerfield 1989, 1998; Peniston Bird and Summerfield 2007). The white non-migrant women who talked to us had varied but often generally good memories. Those who had had to move across the country were on the whole less enthusiastic about the war and the move. One said that she had come up north when her husband came out of the army and moved to work in his father's business.

I came up here. I didn't like it ... I didn't like it one bit, you know. I didn't like it at all. Everything was dirty and so on and the weather ... when I saw the first lot of snow ... and uh that was in 1947 when it was the big snow ... I hated it.

Another woman had moved to Yorkshire as a child with her family when they were bombed out of London in 1940. She also spoke of the snow as 'a little impression that has stayed with me'.

Other women remembered their childhood in the Yorkshire Dales, where they felt relatively untouched by war. But they did talk about rationing and gas masks. One respondent was a Land Army girl who left her family behind to work on a farm. Another had wonderful memories of spending nights on the dance floor. She had been engaged to be married but the war had led her to meet new people and had presented varied opportunities. In comparison, her fiancé seemed boring, so she broke off her engagement and said that this made her feel 'free'. She began working on aircraft maintenance, donning trousers and clambering on aeroplanes. The war made her realize that she could stand on her own two feet, so that afterwards she trained to be a secretary. She remained single, in full-time employment until retirement and had never regretted this decision. Similarly, other women also recalled a lot of dancing and a great sense of independence in their memories of the wartime years. While generally not experiencing the bombings, death and destruction that characterized life in the big cities, they were still party to the privation that took place. However, the war was mainly remembered as a time when customs and norms were changing and when the lives of women were becoming relatively more free. Yet, as documented elsewhere, although the post-war plans for reconstructing the UK envisaged the continuation of women's need to work outside the home, their role in rebuilding home and family life was, in fact, prioritized (Webster 1998). It is little wonder then that the white non-migrant women in this study still associate one major aspect of their identity as being a wife and mother, where they have had partners and children. In this, they share the experiences, although they are different in terms of cultural execution with the other groups in this study.

The significance of racism

Although all the minority ethnic groups in this research spoke about not feeling welcome when they arrived in the UK and gave examples of discrimination and abuse, it was the African-Caribbean women who most graphically described their experiences of racism. Even though Britain had been a haven of relative safety and refuge for many, migration made many of the women to whom we talked into impoverished 'ethnic minorities'. As a 71-year-old Jamaican born participant told us:

> the things that we met when we come to here we didn't have at home. The abuse and the neglect, you know?

Nothing in their earlier lives had prepared them for the experience of racism that many experienced. The women explained how white people preferred to stand rather than sit next to them on the bus, how shopkeepers would put change on the counter, rather than have to touch their hands, how there was an expectation that because they were Black, they could not speak English, how properties with rooms to let often had signs saying 'no blacks, no dogs, no Irish' and how, because they were black, they were told to go back to where they belonged. This came as a huge shock since, as one woman explained, 'we came here because England was supposed to be our mother country and they needed workers' and because their men and women had been involved in the war. Time and time again, the African-Caribbean women we talked to described how they had to 'stick together' in order to survive. For this reason, friendships begun in the early years have continued into later life. Often living in one room, usually with little furniture, sometimes washing nappies in cold water and getting used to having to use a kettle to wash themselves, meant that everyone was struggling simply to maintain the basic elements of daily life. Further, coming from island cultures where women worked, our participants both expected and needed to find employment. This was mostly done in combination with motherhood. Yet, here again, racism intervened. One 75-year-old African-Caribbean woman remembered vividly the problems:

> When the child [grow] I manage to find somewhere to leave them to get a job. I go in the morning to get a job and someone will go after me and get the job

In addition, it was reported that due to racial discrimination, the women were unable to get, what one termed, 'a proper job', unless they were prepared to work in a factory. Despite the fact that some women had trained to be teachers and nurses:

> the qualification in England, it wasn't good enough for the English people, so all these people, instead of studying, they had to get a job in a factory ... or go to night school and get a better job in years to come.

Even at work racism was a common problem. A British Jamaican woman discussed her experience as a worker as follows:

> I didn't get a good reception from X because it was only two Blacks worked there, which is me and my sister. I used to work downstairs but then, when the work is slow, they put me upstairs and the reaction was so

violent. I had to hold the toilet because sometimes I'm afraid to go ... I got even me hair burnt off there ... and the foreman wouldn't do anything about it. He told me the whites wouldn't have me looking down on them. So I was get annoyed and I always prayed to God to help me that I would leave from there and that's where I was so sick, so I left before I retire.

Another African-Caribbean respondent found herself fighting both racism and policies that required children to be bussed to appropriate schools.

And the thing that really get me down when I was here first time was when time for the children to go to school. I used to live in the X area. And where I was living the school was just about five minutes. And I went there to register the child and they said 'No. Can't take the child'. And other people that are not my colour they go there and they get their children in. And I have to travel away from X and go all the way up to Y. I had to take the child on the bus in the morning. And in the day I would be watching the clock to go and pick her up from there to bring her home ... I had three children going to school. Three children going to different places. Out of the way. So I had to be there in the evening to pick them up ... when my children had to go to school they never send them at a school nearby. One of them they away over Y, and different part of Z.

There was an unsung heroism about the clear sightedness of many of our participants who had remained focused on their intention of creating a better life for their families. A Dominican woman, who is 78 years old, had had ten children. She told us:

I have to go and work and push um in a pram, whether fog or whatever because I wanted to [work]. I didn't come here to sit down.

Like the Polish women discussed earlier, the African-Caribbean participants felt that they had been given no help or information during the early stages of their arrival. They felt that they had been treated as outsiders and that despite changes and improvements over the years, this was still the case, to some degree. They were shocked by the conditions in post-war UK and by the racist treatment meted out to them. As one said in response to a suggestion that things had been 'pretty bad', 'not pretty bad, *really* bad. It was terrible'. Yet, despite all this the women can see that struggling against destitution and resisting racism and its associated stereotypes has, in part, given them the strong persona and identities that characterize them today. In particular, they have developed and honed a clear sense of purpose and a determination that the next generations should not suffer the same kinds of hardship as they themselves had done.

Employment and retirement

Women's life course experiences differed across the groups. Most of the Muslim older women and those from Bangladesh and Pakistan, whose English was poor, had not worked outside the home, although some had contributed to family businesses or undertaken homework, mostly in the form of sewing. Similarly, one white rural woman had married a farmer, received no remuneration for this and had no spending money, although they eventually divorced and she set up a successful bed-and-breakfast business. All the women from the other groups had juggled domestic and child-care responsibilities with paid work throughout their lives, with a few being forced to curtail such activities due to their own or their husband's ill-health. The work undertaken has largely been in the following areas: the textile trade; nursing; teaching; home care assistance; factory work; cleaning; auxiliary work in schools; and shop work. Such paid work has been seen as a source of pride and self-identity, either in its own terms or, even if routine or strenuous, because it was contributing to the family welfare and children's futures. One Polish contributor described how she initially had trouble mastering the loom in her factory. After praying to the Holy Mother one night, she had a dream in which she was able to manage the loom effectively. The next day she followed what she remembered from the dream and from then on:

> I had no more difficulty and I didn't change my job. I worked from 1947 to 1985 ... All those years that I have been working on the same job. And I liked it ... I enjoyed it. Of course, there were some very difficult pieces, difficult patterns. But I knew how to tackle it. And I knew how to find out to sort out the difficulty.

A white working class participant who had had five children recounted how she had worked all her life in a variety of jobs, which ranged from making ice-lollies and being a cinema usherette to steam-cleaning and making wedding dresses – which she loved. She said: 'If you wanted to live, you had to work. But otherwise, that's just been my life'. Many other women also made it clear that paid work had enabled them to feed and clothe their children adequately, rather than provide an income for luxuries.

Many of those who had worked in the paid labour force saw retirement as a time of release from hard work. As one African-Caribbean participant put it, 'now is my time to play'. A focus group of two Gujarati and seven Punjabi women laughed when they repeatedly told us 'we are retired'. Further, those living with family felt 'completely retired' because daughters-in-law were taking on the responsibilities of cooking and housework. For a few participants, mainly white, who had had careers, retirement had been a time of adjustment to a loss of status. Some of the participants mentioned how time had shrunk in retirement and that they did not have the amount of time they had expected for leisurely pursuits.

Yet, retirement had very different meanings for our respondents whose life trajectories have determined their access to resources in later life. The necessity to combine domestic and paid responsibilities meant that many had moved in and out of paid employment, some of which had been part time or a combination of full time and part time. Thus, the working-class women of all ethnic groups in particular had little formal entitlement to pensions. This, in turn, meant that in their later lives, they had to rely on other sources of income, be it partners, family or other state benefits. A few of our participants were still in paid employment, although aged over 60, and there were examples of women who had 'kept going' to 67 years and beyond. This was either out of economic necessity or as a means of 'keeping going', or both.

There is also a sense in which retirement seems to mean something different to women than to men. Skucha and Bernard, for instance, have noted that 'women don't retire' (2000: 31). This refers to the idea that for women the boundary between paid work and the home is extremely blurred and that the idea of 'retirement' is itself a gendered concept because it ignores the unpaid domestic, caring and emotional work that older women continue to do. In contrast, men are seen to 'stop' work, although care must be taken not to ignore recent research that has begun to explore the nature of men's roles during retirement (Peat 2004). There is an interesting blurring between work and leisure for women, which continues in retirement. In our study, work was sometimes done for others, as in the case of voluntary work, and there was a great deal of involvement in grandparenting and child care across all ethnic groups. Class and geographical location play a pivotal part here, with middle class women, who tended to live further away from their children, having less of a role in this area. The African-Caribbean, Polish and some of the Asian women in particular were especially involved in their local communities and community centres, organizing activities and providing food. Many of the women who had sewing skills, which they had used in the labour force, are able to utilize these for themselves and others in their retirement. Their more middle class white counterparts were similarly involved in craft and arts work. Some women had become champions, campaigners and advocates, through political or community involvement or through charitable work, for instance taking older people to hospital appointments, visiting nursing homes or organizing English classes for non-English-speaking older women. One participant has organized Bollywood film sessions for older Asian people at a reduced price at the mainstream cinema, which already offered such an English-language film service for pensioners. It is interesting that although some of the participants had taken up learning new skills, only one out of all the interviewees had done this in relation to computing. There was a hunger among many of the minority ethnic community centre groups for more opportunities for learning.

In short, the extent of our participant's activities while 'retired' leads us to question the usefulness of the term, certainly in relation to the diverse group of women at the centre of our study. To reiterate the findings of Skucha and Bernard (2000), when we asked the eight members of one focus group, who had been reporting in detail about the (non-paid) activities of their daily lives, whether women retire, they responded with a chorus of '*no!*'.

Conclusion

Over time the markers of identity change quite dramatically for women. This is particularly so for the migrant women to whom we talked, who had experienced the additional fluidity of changing nationality. They had moved across state boundaries and by doing so had become constructed as 'different' and 'ethnic minorities'. The move had challenged many of their understandings about social life and their senses of who they were. Although still practised, their language, faith, traditions and rituals all ceased to be the 'norm'. Many moved from warm open spaces into small cold surroundings, where they had almost no skill and know how in dealing with the most basic requirements of everyday life, and they were not prepared for the racism that they encountered. Nevertheless, the women whom we interviewed had a clear sense of their own identities and had their own specific forms of hyphenating their earlier nationality or faith with their current citizenship, without feeling uncertain about either. What was important was the social support offered to them by other migrants of the same family, faith, language or culture, which provided them with an anchor and a sense of belonging.

The formation of identities, together with the ways in which they change or develop, are crucially influenced by life course events and by the roles that individuals play across time. They are also affected by the collective experiences of those groups of which they are members. This chapter has examined the issues of gender and aging, ethnicity and nationality, war and migration, racism and employment and retirement because they figured largely in the stories that the women in our study told. However, this is not the summation of the discussion of identities, since other aspects of their lives have exerted important influences too. Feelings of well-being, the aging of the body, the impact of faith and religion and changes in family relationships, such as widowhood and grandparenting, all impact on older women's sense of self, as the research illustrates. These issues are discussed in the following chapters. We next turn to family and kinship networks and older women's place within and experiences of these.

5

Family networks and the moral economy of kin

Introduction

It has been argued that notions of interdependence, mutual support and obligation within families in contemporary Western societies have been eroded during the last decades of the 20th century. Previous norms concerning family responsibilities have declined over time, due to such factors as the weakening of extended family networks, increased divorce, cohabitation, single parenthood and women's increased participation in the labour force (Robertson Elliot 1996). In this context, particular attention has been paid to the provision of care for elderly relatives and the problems that changing family and household structures bring in relation to this. In particular, dual-earner households can no longer undertake the roles that they have played in the past. Since, in Anglo-Saxon cultures, the obligation to care typically falls to the spouse, the daughter, the daughter-in-law and the son, successively, the fact that more women are working makes it difficult for them to perform such duties (Finch 1989; Qureshi and Walker 1989; Finch and Mason 1993; Arthur et al. 2003). However, although this is clearly a major issue, given the current demographic changes that are taking place, there are other forms of intergenerational support that also require recognition. This is because recent research indicates that this support does not simply flow from adult children to frail parents but can also be provided by older people to their children and grandchildren too (Arber and Attias-Donfut, 2000; Arthur et al. 2003; Peat 2004; Brannen et al. 2005). Further, the emphasis in most research

on family obligations and responsibilities has been on white households. Much less has been written about what happens within minority
ethnic groups (Afshar 1989a)

This chapter is concerned with understanding the process of interdependence across generations. It focuses on relations of obligation,
reciprocity and duty. It considers what our participants meant by the
'family' and the particular significance of kin to them. It explores the
role of the moral economy of kin and its part in facilitating the participation of their children in employment. In this context, the moral
economy of kin is seen not simply as a matter of mutual obligation but
also, for many, as a joyful and an empowering experience. Their
commitment to kin provides women both with a sense of effective
power and with a functionality that places them at the centre of the
kinship group rather than on its periphery.

The chapter begins by looking at the relationship between notions of
interdependence, autonomy and reciprocity and what is regarded as
the moral economy of kin. This presents a context for the rest of the
chapter. It then goes on to look at our participants' understanding of
what constitutes family and the significance of kin in their lives. Of
particular importance is the pride and sense of achievement that the
women gain from their children and grandchildren. The next section
looks at the moral economy of kin *per se* in relation to our study,
emphasizing the duties and obligations that older women see to be
important. The chapter then specifically considers the role of grandmothers and its centrality in women's lives. Finally, attention is given
to those, mainly middle-class rural women, whose family and kin are
not proximate. It examines how they actively construct friendship
networks, with the commitment and potential to fill the void that
family is not able immediately to occupy.

Interdependence and the moral economy of kin

There has been a tendency, both in academic research and in the
rhetoric of politicians and policy-makers, to view later life as a time
when people lose their independence and become increasingly
dependent, either on the state or on those around them. Dependence is
often construed in pejorative terms and is associated with having to
rely on others for domestic, physical or personal care and losing the

capacity for self-direction (Arber and Evandrou 1993). However, there has been criticism of the assumption that older people will necessarily become dependent in this way and that independence should be sought at all costs (Arber and Evandrou 1993b; Friedman 1997). As Arber and Evandrou say, '[d]ependence and independence should not be seen as dichotomies, but as part of a spectrum which involves interdependence and reciprocity' (1993: 19). As with the concept of empowerment discussed in Chapter 3, this dichotomy is rooted in a notion of individualistic liberalism that sees normative man (*sic*) as a freely choosing and rational actor, characterized by self-sufficiency and self-reliance (Robertson 1999). Yet, as Robertson indicates, this bears little resemblance to the daily lives of either men or women whatever their age. This is because 'our very individuality exists only as a result of our embeddedness in a network of relationships both private and public' (Robertson 1999: 83). We are all located and live within complex interrelationships of mutual dependence, which she refers to as 'webs of interdependence' (Robertson 1999: 83). Our individualism is dependent in a myriad ways on social, cultural, economic and institutional contexts. These support us and keep us going as individuals, even though we may be completely unaware of this and take it for granted.

For these reasons the notion of interdependence is becoming increasingly important in relation to studying later life. However, two other concepts are also relevant to it. The first of these, autonomy, tends to be poorly defined and is often confused with, and used interchangeably with, notions of independence. However, autonomy refers to being in a position to make active choices and to take decisions about things that affect our lives, both directly and indirectly, even when we rely on others for support (Dunn 1999). Of course, as with independence/dependence/interdependence, the extent of one's autonomy changes in degree and over time and, for the reasons described above, it will never be absolute. Nevertheless, respecting their autonomy was clearly important for the women in our study. Further, even when older people do become increasingly dependant, for reasons of mobility or illness, for example, respect for their autonomy needs to be retained for as long as is possible.

The second concept that is relevant to the idea of interdependence is that of reciprocity. This involves an understanding of people's (conscious and unconscious) views about their obligations to each other and the claims that can be legitimately made in relation to these. Reciprocity may take various forms. For example, it may be relatively 'balanced', where a similar thing to that which has been received is returned relatively immediately (Finch, 1989). However, it can also be 'generalized' (Finch 1989). In this case, there may be either no directly equivalent reciprocation or no expectation of a specific reciprocation at all. Further, what is returned may be delayed, for instance, when parents care for children who then later care for them. In situations, such as the latter, interdependence can tolerate the delay of reciprocity for some considerable time. Additionally, within the overall framework of accepted obligations, a one-way flow for long periods may also be acceptable.

Notions of interdependence and reciprocity, together with that of autonomy, were at the heart of our participants' relationship with both their immediate, and more extended families as well as with their friends. Most of the women spoke about needing to have a sense of 'purpose' in their lives, meaning a clear set of roles and functions to perform. For many, this lay in relationships with family and kin. Respondents divide into those who have family near at hand and those who, through internal migration within the UK due to work or retirement, were separated from family and friends. The former tended to be the first-generation minority ethnic migrants and white working-class women, who had lived in the same vicinity for a lot of their lives. The internal migrants were white women, who were financially better off and living in suburban and rural areas. This meant that they were rebuilding new networks and a sense of purpose and mutual support, for which church, clubs and shared leisure interests frequently offered a basis.

For women whose family was more geographically proximate, their sense of purpose was crucially, although not completely, bound up with their families. The significance of the ties, tasks, obligations and reciprocities that emerged has led us to describe this as the 'moral economy of kin' or exchanges of support within families (Afshar 1989a). The term has most often been used by anthropologists and those involved in development studies (Stack 1974; Scott 1976). It refers to an internal regime of obligation and reciprocity in which family members expect to support others and to receive support in return (Arthur et al. 2003). Although this tends to be implied in most of the ways in which family is conceptualized in Western studies, the nature and significance of what is done is not always made explicit. Here, we wish to emphasize the moral aspect of the commitment, which involves fairness and duty with ideas about emotional, social and cultural bonds. The idea of 'economy' is important because the roles performed and services provided influence household economies, the work that people do, both inside and outside of the household, the resources that are available to them and how these are distributed. The notion of kin is significant also, because, for minority ethic commu-nities in particular, the idea of 'the family' goes beyond those who might be regarded as just 'immediate' members.

Family and the significance of kin

Most of the older women who participated in this study clearly regarded their families as significant parts of their lives. They spoke of them as being 'close', 'happy, 'supportive' and of not wanting to be 'without family'. When speaking about their families most respondents included husbands, since most of them had been or were married, children, grandchildren and sometimes great-grandchildren, sisters, bothers, aunts and uncles, nephews and nieces. They also included sons and daughters-in-law, although this rarely involved other parts of in-laws' families specifically. Some of the Pakistani, Bangladeshi and African-Caribbean women had very large families. The latter in par-ticular talked about their families as 'huge', with one respondent having nine children, 27 grandchildren and 12 great-grandchildren and another ten children (of whom three had died), 22 grandchildren and 21 great-grandchildren. Inevitably, with families of this size, members were dispersed, both across the UK and the world. However, most had some living nearby and they endeavoured to keep in touch with the others through telephone conversations and visits.

The white middle-class women also tended to have families that were more dispersed. They tended to mention fewer of them, mainly children and grandchildren and brothers and sisters. Yet, although contact with family was necessarily restricted, they still referred to keeping in touch and feeling close to them. For most of the other women, however, contact was both frequent and routine. Most of the white working-class women, for instance, saw children and any grandchildren who lived close by at least weekly and often two or three times a week or even daily. One described how she had a grandson of 23 'and he still comes every day'. Another reported that she was lucky with her family because they were in 'constant contact'.

Similarly, both the Polish and the African-Caribbean participants talked about the closeness of their families. One Polish woman described how her children 'visit me always' and how if her daughter, who worked, did not have the time to come in person, then she would ring her mother. Another told us how she had:

> very good children, both of them. And the grandchildren live nearby and I can go and visit them any time I want. So we keep as a family.

An African-Caribbean respondent reported that she saw her three sons and three daughters who lived locally 'every day'. Another described her family as 'very close together' and said that she saw them every Saturday.

Many of the older women in this study were widowed and most lived on their own, although a few were still living with their husbands. However two of the Polish and one of the African-Caribbean contributors lived with an adult child. The situation for the Indian, Pakistani and Bangladeshi women though was more complex. Half of them lived in joint family households, with sons, daughters-in-law and grandchildren and half lived on their own. Of those living with their extended family, a number expressed the view that they were happy with the arrangement and felt supported, cared for and had companionship. For others, however, there were signs that the situation was not ideal. A British Muslim respondent, who had been a widow for 13 years, indicated via an interpreter that her living circumstances were 'OK' but that, when she felt depressed, she had to hide this from her son as the family did not want her to be upset all the time. She said that she did not feel that she had much control over her life, would like to get out more but was not in a position to complain. Another British Muslim, from Pakistan said that although she was happy living with her son and daughter-in-law, it was important for her to keep her 'mouth shut' in order to avoid arguments. A Gujarati Hindu woman, who had also been widowed for 13 years, described how she was not getting on with her daughter-in-law, since there were rows all the time, which were making her very unhappy. She wanted to live on her own but her son would not allow this. She wanted to have fewer family conflicts and to be able to choose what to eat. She felt that if she lived separately, she would actually get more help from her son and daughter-in-law.

In general, those Indian, Pakistani and Bangladeshi women living alone, rather than in joint families, felt that they were supported by their families. A participant, who came to the UK 25 years ago from India and via East Africa, had daily help from her daughter and grandchildren and others reported that family members visited regularly, helping with the shopping, giving lifts and dealing with domestic problems. Some though reported difficulties. One Muslim woman had come from Pakistan to live with her son when his wife died in order to help with child care. When he remarried, she had to move out and, although her son and grandchildren live locally, they do not visit. Another British Muslim woman also said that her children were not very supportive and did not visit very often. Both these women thought that their children were now too involved in their own lives to be able to help them. Other women also indicated that children, who were born and educated in the UK, may well move away from the family environment once they have jobs. As one British Muslim woman, reflecting on the cultural changes taking place, put it:

> The children got their own life. They want to do what they want to do. And when you ask them sometime, they 'no' we are busy. And then you feel upset. I did everything and now, you know ...

An Indian woman commented that people in the UK tended to think that Asian people, especially the elderly, would be looked after by their families. However, there was the problem of young people moving away for work that was 'happening everywhere' and meant that family structures were changing. Another suggested:

> It's the environment. They say it is affecting them as well because they are living in this country.

Another intimated:

> Again, we got different sorts of families. Some like to go out. Some like to stay with their family.

Thus, there are signs of the fragmentation of the joint family situation among some of the women who talked to us, since a number of them were living on their own. For instance, nine out of thirteen Gujarati participants from one particular Hindu centre did so. This fragmentation is particularly the case where enhanced educational and employment opportunities have become important means through which children can access better futures. Achievement and ambition may lead to mobility and the gradual loosening of family connections. Further, the relative smallness of British houses makes it difficult to live as a joint family. Once extended families breakdown, these minority ethnic households begin to behave more like those elsewhere in the population.

Despite all this, many of our women, including those from the Indian, Bangladeshi and Pakistani communities, spoke of their pride in their children's achievements. This was a constant theme across all ethnic groups and, even in the few cases where a participant did not have children of their own, they took pleasure from the successes of nephews, nieces and other young people with whom they came in contact. In fact, most women saw their children's achievements as one of the most important achievements in their own lives. One respondent, an Irish Protestant working-class woman, who had moved to the UK in the 1950s, explained that although child-rearing had been hard, it had been both worth while and important in itself:

Everything is worthwhile when you see a good achievement and always tell them, always tell them, you're proud of them and always tell them you love them. It's not hard to say. It's not being stupid. What can I say? Tell them why not? It gives them that boost it gives them that mum cares, gran cares, it's important.

Two Polish women told us:

We've brought a family. Those sons of ours are doing quite well. Those grandchildren as well, both of them. My granddaughter is studying now. The younger one is doing well at school. What else?

Anyhow, I am very proud of my sons and I am proud that I did achieve what I did because otherwise I would just die with the mill.

Two women from Pakistan said about their achievements:

You haven't got any worry. Like my son get degree. My daughter get degree and I'm hoping my other two children are going to get somewhere. And then you don't worry about them.

If my children are all educated and have nice jobs that is success in life.

The African-Caribbean women also spoke of the things that they had done for the benefit of their families, of their pride in their successes and how these made them feel powerful. For example:

Yes, yes, this is important. Their achievement makes it worthwhile. I'm proud of them. They are good.

Achievement is having three children and to get them off and to be respected by myself and the family. He [sons] didn't get in no trouble with the policeman and he never stole anything from anybody and, then, it's just an achievement. I felt I did something right. I brought them up to understand the value of things and they need to get their life going and they all turn out very well, you know.

Indeed, most of the women saw themselves as the guardians of their kin and worked to secure its survival, morally and economically. The African-Caribbean participants particularly spoke about how, if they miraculously came into extra money, they would give it to their children so that they could pay off mortgages, buy new cars or get out of debt. Some of the contributors were convinced that parenting was the crucial element in saving the futures of the immediate and more distant kin groups. For instance, the Irish Protestant woman cited earlier said:

You learn from your parents and it goes on and on and on. You learn that way. If you learn the bad way then you're going to do the bad. The parents are always responsible for what the children do. If they're good parents, they do the right thing, the children are going to do it. You might get the odd apple if they get in bad company. There for the grace of God I've gone alright. Mine are fine.

Similarly, an African-Caribbean told us:

Oh yes, it's a good thing. You can stand back and look at your children and grandchildren and know what you've put down there and what you teach them and it will still go on when I'm gone.

Such vicarious deferred gratification, whereby the participants across all ethnic groups had struggled to provide for their children and make possible opportunities that they themselves had been denied, was widespread. However, the women also expressed a desire to retain autonomy and control over their lives. For example, one of the Indian respondents, who was 75 and lived on her own, explained that her daughter-in-law used to do everything for her and that she had had to make a deliberate effort to regain control over her life. She described how she now did her own cooking, washing and housework and was able to decide for herself when and how this was done, as well as when to visit friends and go to the temple. This was important because:

> If I didn't have anything to do, I would just be sitting there doing nothing and my body will give up.

An African-Caribbean respondent indicated that:

> I do what I think is right for me ... Now it's my life so I do have total control over my life ... It does give me more sense of security that I can do what I want for me. I have always put everybody first.

Yet, this desire for autonomy, while expressed in positive tones, also had a vicarious aspect to it. In this, most of the women indicated that they wanted to be seen neither as dependent on their families nor as interfering in their lives. As two African-Caribbean women said, for instance:

> I help when I can. I don't interfere. They have their lives and I have mine. I do what I want to do. If I want to stay in bed all day, I stay in bed all day.

> Oh yes, I get support from them but I have to do this on my own, you see. They all have their own life and I don't want to be dependent on them ... I try to tell them I can look after myself.

Similarly, a Polish woman who lives with her son, daughter-in-law and granddaughter told us:

> So it's four of us and thank God I do not push my nose into anything. Whatever they do or buy or sell, I am absolutely not interfere. It's not my business.

Another, quoting the proverb that you make your own bed and have to lie in it, reflected:

I don't expect my children to leave their work and come look after me. But we will see what comes and then we will cope with it.

In a similar vein, a British Muslim, originally from India, said via an interpreter that her main concern for the future was to remain as independent as possible as, 'while she is here, she does not want to be a burden to her family, either emotionally or physically'. Another woman, originally from Pakistan, commented that since her children were all working, she didn't 'want to have to rely on her kids'. Thus, many of the women in this study have gained, and continue to gain, enormous satisfaction from their involvement in family life. They mostly also want to maintain some degree of voluntarism and are aware of the dangers of over-reliance on family members, on the one hand, and of being perceived to interfere, on the other.

The moral economy of kin

We have already seen how the moral economy of kin is based on ideas about family interdependence and the obligations and reciprocities associated with this, which in some cases extend well beyond the immediate kin group (Afshar 1989b). It is also rooted in older women's altruism, as discussed above. For many of the Indian, Pakistani and Bangladeshi women, particularly in this study, familial ties in the extended kin group had been central to securing their well-being at the point of arrival in the country. A 67-year-old Muslim of Gujarati origin told how:

We came to my brother-in-law's. My husband came first and stayed with him and then we came and just stayed there till he found us some work.

Duty was owed to the extended family. Members of the kin group did not so much form alliances, but rather considered themselves to have been born to their duties or made subject to them due to dire circumstances:

He did not have a lot of money or space. But we were family. We just stuck together till things came right ... We couldn't have done it without him.

A similar story was told by a 68-year-old Muslim woman of Punjabi origin:

We came over to my brother. He had a job, was a mechanic and he had a house ... it was a lot of us, and it wasn't easy, but we were happy. He got work for my husband and then we slowly found our feet.

A Muslim woman from Pakistan, who was married at the age of 13 and had her first child at 14 and second at 15, recalled how she and her family had lived with her sister, brother-in-law, brother, sister-in-law and their son. When her sister-in-law was going through a very difficult pregnancy, she ended up looking after the entire family. Such extended family arrangements are still in operation more recently. For instance, a British Muslim woman had arrived from Pakistan 15 years previously when she was aged 60. She and her husband had moved to be nearer their three sons and three daughters 'when they realised they would be alone there' in their later years.

For many of our respondents, the moral duty of kin did not necessarily involve a reciprocal obligation to exchange gifts and services of comparable value, at some future date (Mauss 1966). They saw their kinship network in terms of a safety net that functioned to protect the group overall (Scott 1976; Platteau 2000, 2004). In this context, blood ties and social obligations were essential to maintaining the system (Collier and Yanagisako 1990). For our respondents, the relationships were enhanced by emotional bonds and mutual trust, which protected the survival of the whole kin group (Stack 1974). For the women we talked to, the moral economy was about imparting power and functionality, which, though sometimes cumbersome, was generally seen to be important and rewarding.

The experience of the moral economy of kin goes far deeper than 'the simple idea that one should help those who help him or (in its minimalist formulation) at least not injure them' (Gouldner 1960: 171). The moral economy of kin discussed here may be seen more in terms of Durkheim's notion of the general moral principle, whereby exchange may be unequal, and yet morally and socially binding. It includes the understanding that Scott has of 'the structure of the moral claims' that 'conform with the sense of obligations felt by others' (Scott 1976: 166). In this context, the sense of obligation and duty is backed by the knowledge of belonging, both emotionally and materially (Anthias 2002). Members of the kin group are born into it, remain part of it and owe their identity and, for many migrants, their livelihoods to it. They also have a duty to respect its norms and demands, by abiding to what the group sees as its mores. The kin group organizes its alliances, and sometimes its property and marriages, to enhance its standing and expects its members, young and old, to abide by these requirements (Tapper 1991). In return, members of the group are expected to be able to depend on the protection and support of the kin network, wherever they may be.

The minority ethnic and white working-class women in this study were involved in elaborate kin networks. They contributed to these by cooking, sewing, ironing, performing other household tasks, by taking on quasi-counselling roles, such as giving advice when asked, and in particular by looking after children and taking them to school. For example, a British Muslim woman living in a joint household reported through an interpreter that she:

> helps with the children. She's got one granddaughter living with her and her daughter's got two children and so sometimes, when they come, she helps with those children as well. She does all the housework and the children's sewing and things like that.

A white working-class woman, whose son had been bereaved, bakes for him once a month, making sure that his freezer is stocked up. African-Caribbean women discussed cooking and sewing for their adult children with families. As one said, she 'helps out when she can'. Similar sentiments were expressed by the Polish respondents. One had sold her house, given the money to her son, who had then purchased new accommodation for his mother and his family to share together. She did not see this action as a sacrifice and said that she had arrived at the 'happiest time of her life'.

> I have a person who I love and he loves me. My son. I have him with me together in the same house and somebody I love around me. And every week the pension come for nothing you know. And I live comfortable. . . . I am happy. I help with the cooking – peel the potatoes or help to wash. She wash and I dry, you know. Dusting around, you know.

Another Polish contributor explained in relation to her daughter:

> when she's working I'll probably do some ironing for her because she is a teacher. So she works five days a week full-time. So I probably do some ironing for her when there's a basket for me. Or cook a meal . . . It helps.

On Saturday or Sunday I come and empty the ironing basket. It helps her because remember she is teaching. She has to prepare for school and look after her own children. So if mum comes and irons a few shirts it helps her.

These unpaid activities contribute to the household economy by freeing up time so that adult children, particularly daughters and daughters-in-law, can work or undertake other domestic duties such as shopping, activities that might prove difficult without such support. However, these are seen in terms of duty and of helping out, rather than as making a more formal economic contribution. The idea of 'helping' was a central word in most women's vocabulary. Many of the minority ethnic and white working-class contributors across the board were at pains to stress how difficult it was for their children, who worked hard to look after their own children and pay mortgages. As one of the latter put it, 'It is hard today. It's hard it is today ... So the parents have to work damn hard to keep up to the things they want.' The same woman described how:

If my family's in difficulty and their houses are being done, they come and live with me for a short period of time or whatever it's going to be. And, uh, you know, I think, I think that's the best way to be because this is when we all learn respect for each other. And you realize what your parents have done for you and then you try and do it back for your children, and hope that your children will do the same for you, which, so far, they are doing.

This notion of reciprocity was very much at the heart of the respondents' views of family and they recounted the numerous acts of support that children and/or grandchildren had performed for them, both recently and in the past. These ranged from things such as providing lifts to shops, hospitals and worship, doing the shopping itself, decorating and undertaking household tasks when the women were not able to do these themselves. The relatively small number of women who felt that they were not receiving the support that they needed from family commented on its absence and clearly felt that it put their family in a poor light. Also of interest are the ways in which our participants found the moral economy of kin and the roles that they played within this to be empowering. Here empowerment was experienced, not so much as their having 'power over' the family, but rather as a dynamic process (Rowlands 1997, 1998) that enabled them to have power to make a difference to family life. This, in turn, reflected and regenerated 'the power within' to continue and to appreciate their role as older women within the family and within the community.

The moral and emotional ties of family were reproduced and symbolized in many ways but particularly through the rituals of eating and celebrating together (Peat 2004). Most of the respondents talked about family meals, both as regular occasions and as special events, such as birthdays and Christmas. One white working-class woman recounted how the previous weekend 'all the family, all my children, there were eighteen of us, children and grandchildren and us grand-parents' had been out to lunch together, an outing that occurred 'every two or three months'. An African-Caribbean participant always cooks for her family when they come at the weekend. She said, 'I still say I finish with cooking, but when they come, you know'. Another recalled how on her birthday she had been working at her local community centre and:

didn't have time to do any cooking for my lot and they came (that) night and, um, the first one said, 'I came rubbing my hands all the way and lose the skin off my hands and there's nothing'. Even though I was out, they expect it because they are used to me making things to eat. All sorts, fried fish and all sorts for them.

The Polish women explained how their families still carried on with Polish traditions. For example:

Well at Christmas we celebrate Christmas Eve, not Christmas Day. Christmas Eve is a family holiday really, you know. And all the family gathers at the table [for] our special supper. We have special dishes, usually meatless.

It's a nice tradition, you know, nice and gay. And it's an opportunity for our families to get together. It is not just our nearest family but the extended family as well.

Thus, the familial network is cemented via social as well as by moral and economic activities. Eating and celebrating together serve to reaffirm family ties and relationships and to position individual members within the kin group (Peat 2004). This helps to engender emotional bonds upon which the moral economy of kin is also based.

Despite their very different points of departure, many of the older women to whom we talked retained a firm sense of their obligations and the importance of playing their part in supporting families. In particular, mothering and grandmothering were recognized as lifelong commitments to care, love and providing hospitality. It is to these aspects of their role to which we now turn.

Grandmothering

The fact that many of the minority ethnic and white working-class women in this study looked after children has been mentioned in the previous section as part of the moral economy of kin, which allows parents, especially mothers, to engage in paid employment. However, this discussion did not give sufficient emphasis to the extent of the grandmothering role that some women performed. Looking after grandchildren was an important and regular activity for significant numbers of women. Further, in underlining its functional relationship to the moral economy, the degree to which being a grandmother also gave rise to the emotions of joy, happiness and satisfaction was also underplayed. The women celebrated grandmotherhood as an achievement and as giving them a sense of maturity (Afshar and Ali-khan 2002). For many it was important, not only in terms of its functionality, but also in relation to the creation of a new source of identity and a 'blessing' in itself. A respondent who had migrated from Ireland said:

> I'm blessed with a huge, huge family. I've got two children of my own and five grandchildren and four great-grandchildren. They all come and see me and they're all lovely.

One of the older British Muslim women explained through an interpreter that when she had looked after four of her grandchildren in the past, she had found it to be an enjoyable experience. Similarly, an African-Caribbean participant, describing how her 5-year-old granddaughter had passed a ballet test and her 9-year-old grandson was good at rugby, exclaimed, 'They are good. They give good interest. Ooh, yes! When the kids come to tell you what they were doing, ooh, its great. Its great'. Another said, 'It give me hope for the future, yes, and, um, my little granddaughter now makes me very happy'. Such child care was generally regarded as a pleasure and not seen as a chore.

Time spent caring for grandchildren ranged from the occasional visit to bringing up grandchildren single-handedly; one white working-class woman had raised her grandson from the age of 3 until he was 17 and felt that this had kept her young. There seemed to be different ways in which child care was performed. For some of the women, it occurred on an *ad hoc* basis, when they were called in, sometimes at short notice when an unforeseen incident had occurred. For instance, a Polish woman reported that she provided assistance when it was needed and many women from across the ethnic groups mentioned babysitting with grandchildren, especially when they were younger, sometimes staying overnight. If grandchildren lived near by, they quite often dropped by without any prior agreement being necessary. Some women were invited on family trips and some organized outings for grandchildren on their own account, for example going to the cinema.

For other grandmothers the arrangements were more formalized. Some, again across all groups, were responsible for taking children to school and/or picking them up from it. Others provided support during school holidays. Others were responsible for looking after grandchildren for a certain proportion of a week. For instance, one African-Caribbean respondent looked after her granddaughter for one-and-a-half days and another indicated that she did so for three days a week. A white woman who was 65 years old and who still worked as a cleaner had a number of grandchildren whom she looked after on a rota basis, sharing the job with other grandmothers in the kin network. As she said:

> They [daughters] couldn't go to work without us [grandmothers] helping. So we take it in turn. But it is not that much work. She [granddaughter] is a real good girl.

In fact, some of the African-Caribbean participants were almost professional grandparents. One, for instance, lived with her grand-children and looked after them while the parents went to work. Another was paid by her son to look after her granddaughter. When her husband died, she was forced to think about finding part-time work and her son offered to pay his mother instead of putting the child in a nursery. At first she said that she could not take payment. However, her son pointed out that he would still have to pay fees so that she might as well have the money instead. This was the only example of money changing hands for child care that arose in this study. In their work on grandmothers, Arthur et al. (2003) also found that this was an unusual occurrence, tending only to happen when the grandmother was highly involved in child care and when the parents worked.

Where grandchildren were geographically distant or if contact was less frequent, the telephone was a means of staying in touch. A white working-class woman living on her own said that her granddaughters contacted her regularly by phone:

> You know, she tells me everything on the phone. So I can really help her because she listens to her Nana.

Another described how her granddaughter telephoned her every day when she had flu asking her if she was 'alright'. In addition to providing child care, this grandmother was telling her granddaughter about her life history, including her experiences of the war, exile and migration from Poland. The granddaughter was using the story for a school project and her mother had transcribed all the recorded interviews onto a computer as a legacy for future generations. Other women similarly saw themselves as guardians of the family history, as well as of cultural and religious traditions. They told grandchildren about their own parents and grandparents and about their own childhoods and upbringing, along with wartime experiences. As already described, the Polish women keep the traditional Christmas Eve celebrations and, such is the community's desire to maintain a sense of Polish identity and culture, there is a small Polish school at the local community centre. The women from the Commonwealth of Dominica organize a big dinner party at the local centre to commemorate Independence Day, when they serve Caribbean food and drink. The Muslim women used their time as grandparents to engage the young with religious practices and beliefs. One, whose son had married a 'white' convert, explained:

> All my grandchildren know their nemaz. I sit with them and we read the Koran and I tell them about our religion and our village (in Pakistan). My daughter-in-law usually joins us . . . She is a great cook. She can make perfect chapattis. We work together and we both enjoy it.

Thus, grandmothers are participants in both the production and the reproduction of the norms and mores that influence the kinship group. They help to shape, develop and recreate the differing cultures and histories within which they are located. In this they are active agents in the conceptualization and changing of the customs, habits and traditions that are handed down through the generations.

Despite the women's generally positive views about being grandmothers, however, there were some qualifications in this regard. Although rewarding and enjoyable, looking after grandchildren could also be seen as hard work. In terms of looking after her children's children, an African-Caribbean participant said, 'I've told them I want my life back'. A Polish woman remarked that now that her grandchildren were growing up and fewer demands were being made on her, she had more time in which to please herself. One of the white working-class women, who told us that she really loved her grandchildren coming, also admitted that it could be tiring. Like some of the other women, she found it difficult to say 'no' to requests for help. Sometimes her daughter would ring up unexpectedly to ask if she might bring her children over or if they could stay a little longer than arranged. She always said 'yes', even if 'not feeling, say, a hundred percent'. She said that, 'they don't sometimes think ... they don't think, well are you doing anything Mum?'. Another of the white women observed that:

> You watch them grow and learn things and you know that at the end of
> the day you give them back to their mother. So you have all the fun and
> they have all the work.

A few contributors, especially those who originated from the Caribbean, deliberately refused to get involved with child care. One said that she thought that she had now done her bit and that she 'just wanted to play'. Another insisted:

> Count me out [of childcare]. I looked after my children before and
> occasionally I look after my grandchildren but now it's my time to play.
> I'm at the end of my life and I'm going to play now.

Thus, being a grandmother constitutes a central part of our participants' lives. It provides a set of roles to be undertaken and bestows a particular sense of self to older women. Being a grandmother places the women in a distinctive place within the family and kin network. There they have a pivotal role in maintaining ties across the generations, transmitting links with the past and reproducing cultural and religious traditions. Although a few women expressed reservations about child care and babysitting, they, nonetheless, still fulfilled this symbolic function.

Kin and friendship networks

Most of the women in this study had strong friendship networks. With the exception of a few of the more elderly and less mobile participants from India, Pakistan and Bangladesh, they spoke about these with enthusiasm and pleasure. For the minority ethnic women, especially the African-Caribbean and the Polish, these friendships had often endured over a long period of time and were also frequently supported via meetings at local community centres. These centres also provided a means through which cultural and religious identities could be constantly reaffirmed. Centres based on ethnicity are important in terms of sharing ethnic food, history and experiences and for fostering communal celebrations. In some cases, this was also encouraged by the presence of satellite television from their countries of origin. For the white and minority ethnic women, these social networks existed alongside, and in addition to, those of family and kin described previously. As with the latter, they were clearly also sources of support and satisfaction

For our white middle-class participants, however, particularly those who had migrated to live in rural areas from other parts of the country, alongside the very few in this study who had never married, friendships acted as surrogate kinship networks of support, which were carefully nurtured. Although they kept in touch with family members, some of whom lived hundreds of miles away or even in different continents, meetings were necessarily infrequent and often limited to two or three times a year. This group had had to construct new friendship networks. They remained in contact with friends where they had previously lived but had taken advantage of the opportunities available in their local communities to forge new ties and commitments.

In fact, these participants had gone to extraordinary lengths to become involved in various groups and activities. This was both a deliberate attempt to meet new people and out of a desire to participate in community life. For example, one woman, who was still living with her husband, indicated that they did not have a lot of time to themselves due to the voluntary work that they undertook. She was involved in three voluntary organizations, including the Women's Institute, where she availed herself of the courses that were organized. She described these activities as keeping her busy, her mind active and as a good way of meeting people and making friends. Some of these friendships were now sufficiently strong that they could call on each other in times of need. She told us:

> Yes, I do think that it's important. I do think that it's up to you to go out and join things and, you know, help out. That is the way you make new friends, really good friends. You help to support each other.

Other women also told us how they relied a lot on their friends. For example:

> Yes, my friends are very dear to me and I feel they have done a lot for me, as well. I do rely on them quite a lot

> We consider each other. It's not necessarily that we need to look after each other entirely. But I think we do consider each other. I have a saying. I always say I love my friends as much for their bad points as their good ones and I hope they will do the same for me.

In addition to engaging in activities, such as organizing outings for frail elderly people, dancing, yoga, joining local history groups, taking a sweet trolley to a nursing home, leading walks, involvement in the Town's Women's Guild and the University of the Third Age, along with many others, church and chapel also provided these participants with interests, a sense of belonging and a network of moral and social support. Women told us that they had 'a whole galaxy of friends', 'lots of friends', 'loads of friends' and 'masses of friends'. One woman, a retired civil servant, who had never married indicated that she had many friends:

> When I come to think how many I have in this area (for her recent seventieth birthday party), there were about fifty. So I didn't think that was a bad total ... there are degrees of friendship, of course. To some people you're close. To others it's more of an acquaintance. But, nevertheless, these are the people with whom I share interests.

93

Given the absence of much family living nearby, the women described here had actively strived to construct alternative networks. Married and unmarried alike had managed to establish a group of like-minded people around them who provided companionship and support. Several contributors, for instance, spoke of how, even at this later stage of their life, their confidence had been boosted by friends encouraging them to do such things as speaking in public, organizing events and acting as secretary to local organizations. Their later years had been enhanced by this. Further, it is clear that close friends have a clear sense of commitment to each other. They help each other out now, visiting friends who are housebound, helping with shopping and transport. The expectation is that this will be carried into the future for as long as it possibly can. As one 67-year-old told us, 'we all look out for each other'.

Conclusion

This chapter has highlighted the significance of family and kin networks in older women's lives. At a time when it is common, in some quarters, for people to bemoan the breakdown of family ties, this research indicates that interdependence and close contact between family members is both expected and the norm for many. In this it supports other research suggesting that relationships with the kin group are an important aspect of most people's lives (Finch and Mason 1993; Phillipson et al. 2001). A strong sense of obligation, duty and reciprocity leads us to talk of the moral economy of kin, with older women playing a pivotal role, through child care and doing other domestic tasks, in allowing other family members to work. In fact, being a grandmother was a significant dimension in participants' sense of self and was seen as an enjoyable and rewarding experience in its own right. Although a few contributors were fed up with child care and a small number were too incapacitated to be involved or their grandchildren were grown up, being a grandmother still had a central and symbolic significance. Yet, despite the importance of kin, participants valued their autonomy and were at pains not to interfere in their children's and grandchildren's business unless asked. These ideas of autonomy, often expressed in terms of not wanting to be dependent on their children, and of not wanting to intervene except by invitation, have been noted in other research (Thompson et al. 1990; Bernard and Harding Davies 2000; Peat 2004). They underline some of the complexities embedded in family relationships, since many women across the ethnic groups clearly also expected to receive reciprocal help from children and grandchildren in the future, where they were not being given or did not need that support already.

We have also described how the more affluent women, mainly rural dwellers, kept in touch with family and kin at a distance. Their social network of kin support had been replaced by one based on friendship and they were very actively involved in negotiating and promoting the latter. Notions of obligation and reciprocity within it had had to be evolved, rather than emerging from the 'bloodline', as is the case with kin.

6

Health and well-being

Introduction

It has been argued that the main determinants of well-being and life satisfaction among older women are physical competence, social skills and economic independence (Gannon 1999). However, knowledge and understanding of what actually constitutes well-being remains elusive despite attempts to identify its general components. Among our research participants health was thought to be *the* most important influence on quality of life and well-being regardless of social and ethnic background. Nevertheless, what was regarded as important to good health varied amongst them and was not simply linked to the absence of illness or the physical capability of the body. This highlights the importance of understanding the interconnections between ethnicity, culture, and how women perceive and experience their health and bodies as they grow older. Definitions of well-being and quality of life range from those that focus on specific socio-economic indicators to those that consider a range of social, economic, environmental and psychological issues and their possible impact on life experiences (Smith 2000b).

Within biomedical discourse quality of life has often been defined in relation to different types of illness and clinical advice/treatment. Hence a 'good' quality of life comes to be associated with a disease-free and physically active body. However, more recently a broader-based approach to quality of life has informed policy on aging and health. This developed the concept beyond the narrow biomedical definition to include a range of objective (e.g., income, transport and housing) and subjective, (e.g., happiness, socializing and fulfilment) issues

(Smith 2000b). The World Health Organization's (WHO) definition of quality of life is a good example of a broad-based approach:

> It is a broad ranging concept affected in a complex way by the person's physical health, psychological state, personal beliefs, social relationships and their relationship to salient features of their environment. (Cited in Smith 2000: 6)

In 1995 the WHO launched an aging and health programme that sought to promote a proactive and positive approach to health in later life. In this key components included: life course issues; health promotion; cultural diversity; gender; intergenerational relationships; and ethics (WHO 1998). More recently policy documents focusing on older people have emphasized the notion of 'active aging'. This is defined in the Policy Framework for Active aging (WHO 2002) as participation in 'social, economic, cultural, spiritual and civic affairs'. Here there is a move towards the prevention of illness through 'the adoption of healthy lifestyles' (WHO 2002) based on activity, empowerment and prevention. This is also evident in the National Service Framework for Older People (NSFO) launched in 2001, with its emphasis on the extension of choice and the promotion of independence in later life.

These attempts to move towards a more positive approach to aging represent a challenge to negative views and stereotypes of growing older. Nevertheless, although these developments promote new perspectives on aging and mention ethnic difference, they tend to conceal the considerable cultural variation that exists across ethnic groups, relating to perceptions and experiences of health and well-being.

Further, despite this move towards a more nuanced understanding of health and well-being in policy documents, there remains a tendency to focus on the relationship between aging, ethnic background and structural inequalities as causal explanations for ill-health and poor quality of life. While the impact of material constraint cannot be denied, such an account tells us little about the rich diversity of meaning attached to health, well-being and empowerment in later life. It has also led to the assumption that, with the exception of material factors, health for older women is based on a uniformity of experience. Such a perspective is overly restrictive and tends to omit difference based on ethnicity, culture and migration (Wray 2003; Wray and Bartholomew 2006). The inclusion of these factors exposes the complex character of what constitutes health and well-being for older women.

In this chapter approaches to health, aging and dis/empowerment based on uncritically applied Western (European/American) medicalized notions of health are contested. This includes definitions of health that are based on biomedical notions about the body, which often construct aging as a disease rather than a natural event (Vincent 2003). Negative messages about growing older are frequently a consequence of the medicalization of aging, with its emphasis on physiological decline and increased dependency. Throughout this chapter health is defined in relation to a social and cultural context and changes across the life course. It is argued that diverse life course trajectories shape experiences of health in later life (Hockey and James 2003). As such the connections between previous life events and women's current and future health expectations are also examined.

The chapter is organized into five sections. The first reflects on previous and current theoretical approaches to the conceptualization of health and well-being in later life. The second outlines women's views on the significance of health and the meanings attached to good/poor health. The third examines the impact of previous life events on participant perceptions and experiences of health as they grow older. The impact of changes to the agility and mobility of women's bodies on well-being are discussed in the fourth section. Finally, the concluding section provides a summary of the main empirical and theoretical issues discussed in the chapter.

Conceptualizing health and well-being in later life

Numerous socio-economic, psychological and physical dimensions complexly shape what it means to have good health and feel well in later life. Although a number of psychologically based measures of well-being have been formulated, many of these tend to conceptualize it as needs- or goal-based. This means that the extent to which individuals have their goals or needs met is taken to be a measure of their subjective well-being (Niebor et al. 2005). However, while psychologically based conceptualizations of well-being offer some useful insights, they tend to be based on liberal individualistic notions of agency and empowerment that often emphasize self-actualization and 'the self as the primary agent in the creation of personal well-being' (Sointu 2005: 263). A core assumption here is that people will rationally pursue goals associated with 'well-being' in a proactive manner (Niebor et al. 2005). Such conceptualizations of well-being, with their emphasis on individual agency, often overlook the social factors that shape life choices and opportunities. Instead they tend to assume that people are able to independently control the circumstances of their lives through the powers of mind and action (Wray 2007). They are also ethnocentrically based on Western liberal understandings of autonomy, independence and agency, and it is these that tend to underpin understanding of what it means to be happy, fulfilled and 'well' in British society (Wray 2004).

It is also the case that those factors thought to be associated with good health and well-being are often theorized in isolation rather than as interrelated and indivisible. Such polarized dualistic accounts of either physical/medical or social/psychological aspects have restricted our understanding of health and well-being. In addition, diverse constructions and understanding of health and how these are influenced by differences in ethnic and cultural background and life history often go unnoticed. This is particularly evident in biomedical perspectives, where health is often defined solely as the absence of disease and 'healthy' lifestyle is often based on Western (European/American) notions of self-surveillance and individual, as opposed to collective, empowerment strategies (Rose 1999; Furedi 2004). There has been a shift from the socio-economic environment as a cause of ill-health to one based on individual responsibility, and this is evident in the way that health promotion strategies encourage individuals to take responsibility for their health and well-being (Bunton and Burrows 1995; Hughes 2000). A consequence of this is that ill health is now more likely to be attributed to a personal lack of health maintenance and self-care (Peterson and Bunton 1997).

Another aspect of this is that medical and health promotion advice on changes to lifestyle are assumed to be appropriate to all regardless of cultural difference. This means that the ability to age successfully and healthily has become synonymous with the ability to remain physically and socially active and resist old age (Laslett 1989; Hurd 1999). Thus, aging bodies are more likely to be regarded as a project of the self, which through consumption practices, is able to remain forever youthful (see, for example, Featherstone and Hepworth 1991). Additionally, well-being and good health come to be associated with personal autonomy and control of the body, so that an ill body is perceived to be out of control. This means that older women are more likely to be expected to take responsibility for their health status and be self-reliant, and less likely to be encouraged to use health-care services. It has also had the effect of legitimating a rationing of access to health care for older people (Vincent 2003).

The medicalization of old age, with its emphasis on aging as problem-filled, has shaped societal and individual expectations of health and physical capacity in later life (Vincent 2003). It has also meant that biomedical research, in its attempts to find a 'cure' for the effects of biological and physiological aging, has focused on technological, surgical and pharmaceutical intervention. As a consequence, there is a great deal of medical research that is based on the assumption that the aging body is frail, unhealthy, incapacitated and dysfunctional and needs to be controlled. Through the process of medicalization, aging comes to be associated with physical and mental decline and the need for medical intervention. Some of these medical and technological interventions have benefited older people. However, it is also the case that old age is commodifiable (Vincent 2003).

> Drug companies, finance houses and research establishments have become significant and powerful players in the way our society is organised and in particular for the experience of old age. (Vincent 2003: 142)

In reality this commodification of aging means that the experience of old age now involves self-surveillance and an increase in the responsibility of individuals to maintain a healthy and fit body as they age. This increases the stigmatization of bodily signs of aging in Western culture and creates ever expanding markets for anti-aging medicine and associated commercial products (Goffman 1959, 1963). This has consequences for how individuals perceive their health and the capability of their bodies as they age. For instance, older people often overestimate the dangers of being physically active and underestimate their physical capabilities due, in part, to the contradictory messages they receive from medical science (Grant 2001). Yet there is no clear link between aging and a decline in health and physical capacity; rather, this remains highly contested (Andrews 2001). This is not to argue that bodies are unsusceptible to the passage of time. As Hockey and James note, aging is an embodied process that occurs throughout the life course and which we all share,

> ... be it the onset of menstruation and growth of body hair at puberty, or the wrinkles and grey hair of old age. (2003: 48)

Nevertheless, although changes in physical appearance are read as an indication of aging, the effects of this on individual women are by no means predictable. It is simplistic to assume that all women, regardless of geography, ethnic and cultural identity and other differences, will experience their bodies in the same way. Such a position fails to take account of specific everyday socio-cultural and political practices and how these influence women's perceptions and experiences of their bodies, throughout the life course. It also leads to the often universalizsed assumption that women prioritize appearance over the functionality and capability of their bodies. Significant here is the idea, discussed in Chapter 3, that physical changes to the body mask an inner more youthful self and that an aging appearance is potentially disempowering, posing a threat to identity and well-being in later life (Featherstone and Hepworth 1991; Biggs 1997). This is most apparent in the moralistic imperative to maintain and 'refurbish' bodies, both inside (maintenance of health) and outside (maintenance of appearance). Yet this theory is not based on 'any sustained empirical analysis of older people's experiences', nor is it sensitive to differences in ethnicity, culture, space and time (Irwin 1999: 695). Further, it reinforces the notion of an unchanging 'ageless self' that is superior to the body (Kaufman 1986). This shares similarities with continuity theory and its premise that self-identity remains constant throughout later life, despite visible bodily changes. Such an approach is problematic because it upholds the mind–body dualism and the assumption that the body is simply a tool of the mind (Grosz 1994). Positioning mind and body as distinct spheres has the effect of reducing the body to either the product of the mind (intellect and reason) or the product of experience (the sensual and unreasonable). This means that the complexities of the relationship between the two spheres are rendered invisible.

Despite this we know that bodies are carriers of history, status and identity and represent 'all of past and future gathered up in the present' (Adam 2004: 101). Body and self are closely interrelated as changes to our appearance and the physical functionality of our bodies continuously disrupt our perceptions of self and identity (Hockey and James 2003). In her discussion of women's empowerment and embodiment in later life, Morell argues that it is not possible to control the health of the body to 'order'.

> When we understand that the body is not controllable, those who cannot control their bodies will no longer be seen as responsible for their limitations or as examples of 'unsuccessful aging'. (2002: 10)

But this message is often at the centre of biomedical and health promotion discourse, which acts both as public educator, aiming to enable individuals to make informed health choices, while simultaneously serving as a 'refined and pervasive system of control' (Lee and Jackson 2002: 125). This medical system of control, with its emphasis on self-surveillance, means that health-care policy and practice is inclined to focus on prevention rather than intervention. For older women, the subtext of this message is that aging is a preventable disease that can be managed through self-surveillance. It is not surprising then that in her research on how women negotiate health issues, Hurd (1999) found that women actively resisted the identity category 'old'. In order to do this they defined themselves in terms of 'activity' and 'independence' and viewed 'health problems as minor inconveniences that must be overcome' (Hurd 1999: 430). Additionally, women who defined themselves as 'not old' were more likely to manage their health through practices of self-surveillance and prevention.

Practices of self-surveillance within biomedical health discourse are constructed as empowering because they enable women to resist aging through diet, exercise and other regulatory devices. The underlying premise of medical discourse is that good health can be achieved through self-education and surveillance. A side-effect of this is the stigmatization of illness and those who become ill, and the association of independence, activity and good health with successful aging, and dependence, inactivity and illness with disempowerment and a lack of status. This sends out a clear message to older women; they must resist illness in order to maintain their status and agency. This is evident in Hurd's (1999) research where the women are so threatened by this stigmatization that they instead keep their health fears to themselves and define themselves as 'young-old'. Williams and Barlow also note this type of resistance in their research on the effects of arthritis on lay perceptions of the body. As they suggest:

> ... bodily changes fuelled feelings of self-consciousness particularly when in contact with strangers and current or prospective partners, provoked feelings of being different and highlighted fear of stigmatisation. (1998: 138)

The effects of ethnic and cultural identity complicate this further. Culturally specific norms and taboos govern bodies in different ways. Vom Bruck (1997) argues that Yemeni Muslim women's bodies are culturally defined according to moral codes and practices. Specifically, the body is not communicated, 'it must not be seen, smelled, heard or touched' (Vom Bruck 1997: 179). This contrasts with Western moral codes and practices that define women's bodies as visible and the 'object and prey' of men (De Beauvoir 1970: 642). Hence, older women's perceptions of health, physicality and the significance they attach to their bodies are marked by cultural diversity. Therefore, it is important to understand the complex relationship between ethnic and cultural identity, the lived reality of a body that is aging and how these connect to experiences of health and well-being.

Cross-cultural gerontology has focused on aging in relation to the experiences of ethnic minorities and the migration of older people (Torres 1999). Within this, research on health and ethnicity has explored ethnic variations in health and illness and the link between ethnicity, inequality and health (Markides 1989; Keith et al. 1990; Blakemore and Boneham 1994; Karlsen and Nazroo 2002). There has been a tendency to focus on material constraint, service provision and the types and rates of illness linked to specific ethnic groups (see, for example, Blakemore and Boneham 1994). This has meant that the relationship between age, ethnic identity, embodiment and health has often been overlooked. Further, these accounts often concentrate on the health experiences of older men, so that women's experiences frequently remain hidden or are referred to briefly. Consequently, little is known about how ethnically and culturally diverse backgrounds shape *women's* perceptions of their health and well-being as they grow older. More emphasis on the cultural context of women's experiences of health and aging may provide alternatives to dominant Western biomedical perspectives of what constitutes good health in later life.

Health and well-being: different perspectives

Our participants were asked how they felt about their bodies and health, as they grew older. A number of women spoke of health problems and how they could potentially interfere with the quality of their lives. Illnesses that caused most concern were those that impacted upon the functionality, agility and mobility of their bodies, such as arthritis, broken limbs, asthma and diabetes. For the majority, good health formed a major component of happiness and well-being, which generated feelings of agency and empowerment.

> Good health that's all I'm asking for because there is no point having a house full of money and the health is no good. (African-Caribbean woman, aged 65)

> That [health] is the most important thing in my life. Good health. If one hasn't got good health you're nowhere. It is very, very, important to me good health. (Black/West Indian woman, aged 61)

> Well I just hope to continue being healthy, I think that is the main thing and just carry on as I am now really. (British woman, aged 68)

Most of the women saw good health as a central component of well-being and often more important than income and other material factors.

> If you've got your health, you've got everything. I think if you've got your health you've got wealth ... I think so, I mean, yes, if I can keep my health that's my main worry. (English woman, aged 65)

> Well I think if I am healthy life, then life, won't be hard. Because I can go any place I want. I don't need to stay at home. Always at home stay by myself, because healthy people they can go everywhere, poorly people and old people they just stay at home in a chair. So I think it is more important our health if we get proper medication. (British/Polish woman, aged 72)

> Well if you were not as healthy as you were you wouldn't be able to do

the things that you want to do which is your quality of life really isn't it? (British woman, aged 68)

These quotations capture the significance of health for other areas of life such as activity, socializing and avoiding the negative stereotypes associated with aging. An agile body that is able to carry out the actions and movements necessary for participation in social life is important, because being with others is intimately connected to the maintenance and construction of social selves, identities and networks (Goffman 1971; Hockey and James 2003). The way in which we control and present our bodies in everyday social encounters signifies who we are, and what we are capable of, to others. However, this does not mean that ill-health and/or physical conditions, such as arthritis, prevent women from being social, active and enjoying life. Instead resistance to changes in the physicality and functionality of the body is ongoing and occurs throughout the life course.

When asked what good health meant to these women, they summed it up in different ways. For a majority of them it was directly linked to the presence or absence of illness and the pain and discomfort associated with this. When speaking about the health of their bodies, women tended to use mechanistic biomedical terminology, with some referring to medicalized accounts of their health status rather than their own lived experience of it.

> ... My doctors' always saying, 'you should go out' because I've got arthritis and I have diabetes and, um, high blood pressure I suffer from. And also osteo-arthritis, all these things. (Ugandan woman, aged 58)

> She's saying she went to the doctor to see him about the arthritis and she explained that she got pain. He said 'well at your age it's not going to go. There's no cure for it. It's only going to get worse' (Translator, focus group with Pakistani and Indian women)

> And she gets told by her own GP that it's because of her old age, the health problems. (Translator, focus group with Pakistani and Indian women)

In these quotations, the negative views of aging bodies held by the medical doctors involved resulted in women receiving inadequate health-care advice and provision. To be told that health problems are simply a consequence of aging is unhelpful and misleading. It is perhaps not surprising that a small number of women turned to alter-native remedies, often passed from generation to generation, to combat health problems. For instance, one 71-year-old British Jamaican has arthritis and high blood pressure and uses 'home remedies' to improve her health:

Do you feel the treatment from doctors has been okay? (Interviewer)

Well all I get is some tablets. But I try ... you have to try a home remedy because sometimes ... they say garlic tea is good for arthritis.

And cod liver oil? (Interviewer)

Well I don't like the cod liver oil. I used to take the tablet but it don't let me feel ... it upset my stomach. Yeah, but the garlic tea, it's good. When I do it I just squeeze a bit of lemon you know to take away the taste [...] You know, because I used to visit the doctor so often an' now when I go he says my blood pressure is not bad.

This participant supplements traditional Western medicine for high blood pressure with garlic tea, a credible 'home' treatment. When referring to 'home', she is speaking of Jamaica rather than England. Hence, her use of alternative remedies connects her to a homeland and a collective ethnic/cultural identity and tradition. How women inter-pret the health of their bodies and respond to Western biomedical advice and treatment is bound up with past and current ethnic and cultural belief systems and values. This means that individual and collective histories of culture, ethnicity, religion and space influence women's responses to their aging bodies and the significance they attach to Western biomedical approaches to health and aging.

Rather than being linked exclusively to physical criteria alone, the meaning of good health was complex. This is evident in the following points made by Indian participants:

Good health is when you are happy, physically and mentally healthy. (Indian woman, aged 62)

Generally I have enjoyed good health. For the past six years I have had knee problems, which causes discomfort in my walking. Good health is having the mind, soul and physical free from foreign diseases. (Indian woman, aged 62)

In these examples mind, soul and body are interwoven so that good health is not simply related to the physical body. Moreover, all of these are depicted as possible sites of disease.

In our research, health and well-being were also linked to family and friendship relationships, religious and spiritual belief and the formation of social bonds with others (Afshar et al. 2002). Attachments to others through shared activities, interests or participation in conventional everyday tasks create social ties that connect older women to wider society. This is significant because it becomes more difficult for women to maintain membership of a social group or network if they encounter changes to their mobility or health. For our participants, changes to physical health were defined as potentially problematic if they were likely to interfere with 'keeping going' and being able to carry out everyday tasks:

> ... your health is most important because there are so many things you can do if you have health. But obviously, if you haven't, you are going to be limited and then it takes a lot of courage and initiative to change and adapt and adaptability is a lot more difficult when you are older than when you are younger. (English woman, aged 67)

> Well good health means a lot to me because you can get up and go. Not depending on anybody, you can do what you want for yourself. You can clean your teeth ... I can get up and go. I can always help somebody else. (West Indian woman, aged 64)

These participants emphasize the importance of being able to move around and 'get up and go' to achieve both independence (autonomy) and interdependence (reciprocity – helping others). In these accounts mind and body coexist so that changes to physical functionality may disrupt the construction of social selves and identities (Hockey and James 2003). This may be due to problems with physical mobility, which restrict participation in social events and opportunities to interact with others. As the previous English woman points out, changes to health may constrain choice and opportunity and create limitations to which is is difficult to adapt. Women need to be able to continue to undertake routine tasks, interact with others and take on social roles and responsibilities, because these are central to the creation and continuation of individual and social identities. As such the continuation and development of interdependent relationships and opportunities to fulfil social roles are important to women's happiness and general well-being.

An essential ingredient of health and well-being for all our research participants was the opportunity to form and maintain relationships with others. These links between health, well-being and family and friendship networks have been noted in previous research (see for example, Jerrome 1981 and Jocelyn-Armstrong 2000). Spending time with family generated feelings of good health and well-being, as these Indian women explain:

> This lady says, actually, when her children visit her and she feels really happy. It's healthy for her. (Translator, focus group with Indian women, age 70+)

> *Interviewer*: Would you describe yourselves as being in good health?

> She says, 'Its okay as long as I'm getting on with my life'. She's happy because she got a good family and they visit her and feel happy about it. If you feel happy, you feel healthy as well. That's what they are trying to say. What she is trying to say is the relationship as well. The family. If you've got a good relationship you feel healthy as well. Yes it's the relationship actually. That does make health. (Translator)

Social companionship and attachment to others create a sense of belonging, confirming identity, status and role. Hence, for these women a 'good relationship' with family members contributed to their physical and mental health and well-being.

Embodied health experiences: connecting past, present and future

Life histories and cultural ideologies together influence women's expectations of the capabilities and possibilities of their body as they grow older. Earlier embodied experiences are 'gathered up in the present' so that previous incidents extend into and influence, present and future (Adam 2004: 101). Yet this process is by no means linear; rather, it is disordered and produces a diversity of effects that may or may not influence women's current and future health experiences and priorities. Hence, the effects of previous embodied life events, for example, poverty, discrimination, migration, cultural regulation and illness, are literally written onto the body and have consequences for women's health and well-being (Wray and Bartholomew 2006). Such occurrences may, for instance, create susceptibility to restrictions in physical movement or activity or have detrimental effects on women's confidence and sense of self. It is not possible then to separate past, current and future time and space when conceptualizing experiences of health and embodiment; rather, these are interlinked (Adam 2004). This is evident in women's accounts of their past and present life experiences and what health means to them. For some women previous life events and the materiality of time and space continue to shape their current lives and their mental health. As two Bangladeshi women noted:

> ... when I was young I had too many responsibilities to feel young. I cared for my brothers and sisters and now my own children ... I am not in good health. I have been mentally ill for some time. Feeling tired all the time. (Bangladeshi woman, aged 58)

> I have not been able to socialise with people in England. They live different lives than Bangladeshi. I cannot read or write I had good health all my life but I feel depressed. I was told by the doctor I need to go out and socialise more. I am in the house 90% of the time. (Bangladeshi woman, aged 61)

Gendered socio-cultural expectations and life events such as migration influence the type of role women take on across the life course and the timing of embodied experiences and rituals, such as marriage, parenting, grandparenting and retirement. For some these roles and events continue to shape the responsibilities they have and the space they inhabit as they grow older. The first Bangladeshi woman above speaks of 'too many responsibilities' and how these have shaped her past and present life and health. She felt old when she was a young age and does not feel that she has good health. In particular, she feels that her mental health is poor. For the second woman past experiences of migration and her present feelings of isolation are inseparable. Although she has good physical health, she feels depressed because she is not socializing with others, but instead is spending most of her time in the house. As such, good health is not linked to physical criteria alone but is also related to active involvement with others (Afshar et al. 2002). In both of these examples past and present experiences connect, influencing the women's health and mental well-being and the opportunities available to them (Adam 2004).

For other participants, childbearing, wartime experiences and past illnesses had not been forgotten but continued to influence their current health and happiness:

> After having nine children my health is very poor. (Pakistani woman, aged 59)

> I have bad back always because I was in Germany during the war working and it stays forever. (British/Polish woman, aged 72)

> I was told when I was eighteen I had bronchitis because I always had a little cough because I had pneumonia three times which is why I failed my medical for college. I was told I would have to live with it for the rest of my life but I have never let it worry me. I am always aware I have a cough. Sometimes it is fine especially if it is lovely weather, but sometimes it plays up a bit ... (White British woman, aged 67)

Embodied memories such as these are written onto women's bodies simultaneously, reminding them that they are aging and that they have lived through traumatic life-changing events. This was also the case for a contributor who had undergone a mastectomy 20 years previously and felt healthier as she grew older:

> ... I actually feel more healthy now than I used to when I was younger because, of course, you don't have period pains so that's not ... I don't have PMT each month. I feel energised in a way by being older and being free of women's complaints. In fact, I even carelessly lost a breast 20 years ... so even half a bit of my femininity went as well [laughs ...] Well, having had a mastectomy, which is quite a shock to the body, you know, in a way nothing else after that matters. If your skin ... your thighs get a bit saggy or whatever nothing matters. (White British woman, aged 60)

In these examples past and present experiences of embodiment overlap and are interconnected so that 'to be *in* the body is to be in time' (Game 1991, cited in Adam 2004: 56). Our bodies provide a link to the past as previous events and transitions are written onto the body and serve as a continuing reminder. For instance, giving birth to nine children continues to affect our previous Pakistani woman's health as does the war work undertaken by the Polish respondent, which means she has a 'bad back'. Similarly, the white British contributor notes how the illnesses, which she suffered in her youth, have left her with a cough that still 'plays up a bit'. In these examples the health of women's bodies and their well-being is not simply related to present events and circumstances. Instead, past incidents extend into the present and future and have a continuing effect on the health of women's minds and bodies and how these are negotiated in later life. The impact of cultural norms and values, historical events, and previous illnesses are written onto the body and do not simply disappear with the passage of time (Wray and Bartholomew 2006).

Being *in* the body: embodiment, health and physical activity

Women negotiate and resist health issues and problems throughout their lives and as such this is not simply a feature of later life. Responses to illness or changes in physical agility varied among our participants in relation to previous interests and opportunities. For some participation in exercise and physical activity promoted a sense of achievement and well-being. It was also a means of resisting changes to mobility and agility that occur throughout the life course.

> I have always liked exercise. I used to play a lot of sport. When I had to give that up, I sort of went on walking. I love being out in the fresh air. I like the achievement. Sometimes it is painful getting up the top of these hills but it is a real sense of achievement. (White British woman, aged 61)

> I get aches and pains sometimes, but, you know, I go to the gym and try to keep fit ... This morning I was there at seven. (Black West Indian woman, aged 61)

> I can't run, that's one thing I can't do since I broke me knee. I can't run but I can dance ... if there's dancing, I mean, I'm up dancing all day you know. (British/Irish woman, aged 66)

Through physical activity these women resist aches and pains and changes to the physical capability of their bodies as they age. Physical activity also provides women with opportunities to move and exert their bodies and act out social identities. In this respect the women quoted above are not simply resisting changes to the physicality of their bodies. They are also constructing and renewing particular social identities that generate feelings of agency. In this body and self are closely entwined so that the acts of 'doing' and 'being' become inseparable. For example, the British/Irish respondent constructs an active embodied social identity through 'doing' when she dances. This, in turn, provides opportunities to exist and engage with others.

However, if 'doing' becomes more difficult, women do not necessarily disengage from activity but instead negotiate new ways of remaining active. For instance, a West Indian participant, aged 64, views this as 'slowing down' rather than 'being ill':

> In general it [body] is slowing down and, um, you know there are things you could do and you can't always do it. You can do it but you do it at a slower pace. I couldn't get up and clear the house, top to bottom like I used to do. But I know I will do upstairs on one day and another day I do the downstairs ... It's got its set-backs but it's not being ill.

This participant lives with her body, rather than simply inhabiting it. She adapts to its ever changing rhythms. Her 'self' is neither ageless nor disconnected from her body; a more youthful self/mind does not act over her body and control its functionality to order (Morell 2002). Yet the assumption that it is both possible and desirable to maintain a 'youthful' body prevails and is central to Western health promotion, medical discourse and notions of successful aging (see, for example, Biggs 1997 and Laslett 1987). In this message individual responsibility for health is uppermost, so that good health is associated with high levels of physical activity and poor health with a less active lifestyle (Hughes 2000). The above respondent, however, does not concur with this because she insists a slower pace of movement and activity is not the same as 'being ill', a label that she resists (Hurd 1999).

Nevertheless, some women had become less active due to health-related problems and this left them feeling frustrated. In a focus group held at a sheltered housing complex, one white English woman reflected on how Parkinson's disease had gradually curtailed her friend J's ability to dance. Her friend joins in the discussion to comment on how this had interfered with her sense of self.

> You see I'm going to give an example here with you, J. She used to go dancing twice a week and go out walking and then she started with Parkinson's disease, so it has curtailed her interests a lot. (English woman, aged 63)

I go [dancing] to watch but I get mad because I can't get up and do it with them, you see … I can't do it anymore. They ask me to go and I do a bit and say 'I can't do it' and they say 'course you can'. But I get all worked up. They all say 'are you alright?' They feel sorry for you. You might as well sit at home than sit three hours doing nowt. So is it me or am I being funny? (J, aged 64, English)

Interviewer: I think it must be awful if you have to sit and watch something that you want to do.

That's it you see … You're still sat while everybody's … good luck to them. I mean, I used to enjoy doing it but you just feel nagged and you just want to get up and do it. But you can't turn around. You've got to wait until that feeling comes into your feet. Then you can move that's what your sticks for you see. You've just got to make the best of it love. (J)

This contributor is watching rather than doing and this leaves her feeling isolated from her friends, frustrated, self-conscious and ultimately disempowered. Having a degree of control over the body and its capabilities is bound up with feelings of autonomy and power, particularly in Western society. To be seen to have control over the body, rather than being controlled by it, signifies capability, independence and autonomy to others. This means that J is encouraged by her friends to maintain a degree of control over her body by continuing to dance even though she struggles with this. As a consequence she feels 'nagged' and finds her loss of mobility disempowering. J risks stigmatization if she does not resist her illness, as others interpret this as 'giving in' to the body. This is read as disempowering because it is associated with lack of control and loss. Since Western conceptualizations of agency and empowerment prioritize autonomous action and independence as essential to well-being and successful aging, it is not surprising that J's inability to continue to dance independently and maintain control over her body is constructed negatively by others (Wray 2004). Dance and other activities were generally associated with a youthful identity. This is apparent in the following example:

… I go dancing a lot, so I don't feel old when I'm dancing because I love it. So that helps to keep me feeling young. (White British woman, aged 60)

113

This participant is using physical activity to construct and communicate self-identity. When she dances she feels young because she is able to express her self through her body. Her experience of dance is embodied. This is not to say that her experience of dance is simply the performance of a more 'youthful' identity, or that her body somehow conceals a more youthful self (Featherstone and Hepworth 1991). Rather, it is to argue that the physical functionality of the body, rather than its appearance, is a significant indicator of well-being. Dance is also a communal act that places this contributor in close relation with others and this communicates a variety of meanings, as Frank suggests:

> Dyadic relation with others who join in the dance implies an associatedness which goes beyond one's own body and extends to the body of other[s]. (1991: 80)

Dance then facilitates physical and social contact with others and sanctions a type of shared intimacy that is often absent from other aspects of everyday life. The inseparability of mind and body are also confirmed as biological, psychical and social dimensions of experience, which combine to produce the personal well-being described by our previous respondent.

Conclusion

This chapter set out to examine the health and well-being experiences of older women from diverse social and ethnic backgrounds. It has problematized Western biomedical approaches that through scientific legitimization have constructed aging as a disease and medicalized the process of growing older. Central to this is the argument that this biomedical discourse often has negative consequences for how women view their health and the capability of their bodies as they age. As noted earlier in this chapter, it was common for our participants to rely on medical terminology to describe their health and well-being. Additionally, when describing what health meant to them, the absence or presence of disease was often regarded as a key indicator of health status. Medical science has identified aging as a health problem, so that growing older is routinely linked to ill-health and risk. There is an expectation that poor health or some degree of immobility will always accompany aging. As being able to 'get up and go', 'help others' and socialize were priorities for our participants, it is not surprising that they cited good health as the most important indicator of well-being.

A further issue raised in this chapter, and often absent from current conceptualizations of health, is the impact of previous life events on present and future expectations and experiences of health. When considering present health and well-being, a number of our participants reflected on their life histories and the lingering after-effects of the events and traumas they had lived through. This was often the case for migrant women who, through geographical movement, had experienced separation from friends, family and culture. For some, particularly Bangladeshi women, this had a long-lasting impact on their health and well-being as they grew older in an unfamiliar society and culture. They spoke of their isolation and the impact of this on their mental health. This was the case for one respondent who, though in good physical health, felt depressed and rarely left the house.

The gendered nature of the life course powerfully affects women's life experiences and subsequently their health and well-being. However, the way in which gender is constructed varies across culture, time and space. Hence, women's life trajectories are gendered in different ways. Thus, cultural values and norms may limit the range of possibilities and options available to women throughout their life course and alter the timing of major life events. For instance, the timing of childbirth and marriage creates different perceptions of what it means to be young, mid-life and old. This is clearly evident in the accounts of Pakistani and Bangladeshi women, who were more likely to describe themselves as 'old' at an earlier age than other participants. Cultural norms and values that construct the role of women differently permeate the symbolic meanings attached to motherhood, marriage and growing older.

A central argument of this chapter is that older women's health and well-being cannot simply be reduced to social and material factors or to biological aging alone. Rather, the ways in which women perceive their health and experience their body as they grow older is complexly linked to a number of factors such as culture, life history and individual priorities and expectations. Dimensions of time, space and location overlay these. Thus, there is a need to develop an approach to health and aging that is sensitive to diversity and the connections between previous life events and current and future health expectations and experiences.

7

Faith and identity

Introduction

Religion has generally been ignored as a resource for older people, in this case older women. Even though patriarchal religions have been criticized as being oppressive to women, the majority of believers are nevertheless female, who are the main transmitters of tradition (Cornwall 1989; Batson et al. 1993; Franks 2001b). When directly asked, 'What is the most important aspect of your quality of life?', religion was not offered as *the* primary ingredient by the majority of our respondents. Nonetheless, faith was integral and frequently central to the lives of the greater number of them and was often linked to health (Coleman et al. 2002). Readiness to talk about faith was especially marked in the case of first generation migrant women, who attributed many quality of life outcomes, including health and well-being, to their faith. Clearly then religion is an aspect of ethnicity that needs to be taken into account in constructing a culturally sensitive and appropriate theoretical framework for the study of aging and empowerment (Torres 1999).

In this chapter various aspects of our participants' religious beliefs and linked practices are discussed. It shows that for the older women in our study, faith is not solely a black or a minority ethnic issue. It is also a matter of importance to many older white women, who may also engage in spiritual and religious practices as a cornerstone to their lives. Further, the faith discussed by all the women is not narrowly confined to attendance at formal acts of worship, but involves activities and ways of communing with their gods. The chapter begins by providing a context for what follows, offering an introduction to the ways in which religion is currently being debated and issues around secularization. It goes on to examine the relationship between religion and aging, faith and identity, and ideas about reflexivity and spirituality in relation to our participants. Following this there is a discussion of some of the positive contributions that respondents reported that faith has brought to their lives. This focuses on its social benefits, the significance of prayer and the role of pilgrimage. The chapter then looks at some of the difficulties that older women reported, focusing on doubt and how they are sometimes excluded from formal and more informal forms of worship. It concludes by reiterating the centrality of faith and the need for it to be taken into account in understanding and analysing the aging process.

Ways of thinking about religion

The main thrust of the study of religions in academia has been from a secular viewpoint. Hangraaf defines religion as 'any symbolic system that influences human action by providing possibilities for ritually maintaining contact between the everyday world and a more general meta-empirical framework of meaning' and 'a religion' as the latter 'embodied in a social institution' (Hanegraaff 1999: 147). The first definition spills over into the notion of 'implicit religion' (secular practice that contains unspoken embedded religious aspects), and the second, not only to obvious examples of organized religion, but also 'civil religion' as well as 'cultural religion' Both within and around the 'borders' of organized religion, there are the concepts of 'spirituality' and 'personal spiritualities'. As King suggests, spirituality can be understood as 'wider than religion', on the one hand, and, on the other, as 'the deepest and most central part of religion' (King 1996: 219). It can also theoretically be outside the parameters of religion (Hanegraaff 1999: 151). Hanegraff defines a spirituality as 'any human practice which maintains contact between the everyday world and a more general meta-empirical framework of meaning by way of the *individual* manipulations of symbolic systems' (Hanegraaff 1999: 147). Spiritualities then, as opposed to spirituality within organized religion, are personal forms of belief that slip outside of the boundaries of traditional faith communities and incorporate the beliefs and activities of non-practitioners of explicit faith systems and those who do not embrace scientific rationalism alone. Spiritualities fit with liberal and individualist cultures. Durkheim recognized the potential for this kind of privatized religion – religion as it were of one believer instituted by that believer (Durkheim 1995: 42–44). This is a concept very much in keeping with a postmodern age.

Organized religions are not homogenous, because springing from the various religious traditions, there are not only revivalist forms of religion but also new religious movements, New Age or 'popular religion', as well as new organized spiritualities frequently, but not always, deriving from 'traditional' religions (Sutcliffe 2003). Although it is usually expected that new religious movements and personalized forms of belief will be more attractive to younger people, there is some evidence of elements of New Age beliefs and individual spiritualities in our study. New spiritualities that draw eclectically on older faith systems may offer opportunities for women, who may find themselves unable to fit the requirements of mainstream religious organizations, through marriage outside the group, sexual orientation, cohabitation or remarriage.

In these kinds of circumstance, a way of coexisting with one's faith without rejecting it has been identified by Davie (1994). She refers to this as the phenomenon of 'believing without belonging', believers who do not actively participate in organized religion but who accept a privatized form of spirituality and its dislocation from public religious life. The phenomenon of 'believing without belonging' is eclectic and extremely difficult to categorize. It is quintessentially postmodern (Wright 2000). This has emerged as the case particularly with participants in this study who were disillusioned with congregations. A white rural participant said:

> I realised I just couldn't stand it any more, people grumbling about who was singing in the choir. I thought well really this is just ridiculous

Another white rural participant, aged 61, said, 'I feel closer to God out on the hills'. Participants who fell into the 'believing but not belonging' category tended to be in the younger age range, white and non-migrant. Nevertheless, a Dominican participant also fitted this category:

> My belief is trying to treat people as I would like to be treated myself. I

believe in if you do good it comes round to you. And if you're a horrible person its going to come round as well. But I don't know too much about church.

As suggested above, faith communities are not monolithic and, in general, within the context of British society, there is an age divide in terms of the ways in which faiths are practised. In terms of Islam, for example, Islamic renewal tends to appeal to young (often British-educated) Muslims, who interpret the forms of religion followed by their elders, who are first-generation migrants, as 'cultural religion' marked by customs and cultural accretions, which the young revivalists have deemed to be oppressive (Franks 2001b; Afshar et al. 2005b). 'Customs' are here meant to mean the cultural and social practices of the various South Asian communities, which the first-generation migrants brought with them and which have been practised, modified or intensified since they have lived in the UK. One such custom is that in South Asian families, Muslim women pray at home. However, in her study of young Muslim women in Manchester, Lyon found that the younger revivalist women went to the mosque and listened to sermons in Arabic (Lyon 1995: 51). The separation of the religion, Islam, from a particular culture is important to the young women, because in their view it is cultural practices that oppress them and Islam that is seen as liberating (Franks 2001b, 2006). This is common to revivalist forms of different faith communities and is a means of implementing change, for instance in claiming the Islamic right to choose a marriage partner and, therefore, resisting an unwanted arranged marriage. Other young people may reject their elders' faith altogether, or for a time. Further, there is clearly a diversity of young Islamic revivalists who are from different ethnic backgrounds, including white converts to Islam (Franks 2000, 2002).

Secularism and secularization

Weberian secularization theory and Durkheimian and post-Durheimian re-enchantment are two ways of looking at the status of the secular and the religious. It is only recently that secularity with its perceived neutrality has begun to be interrogated. What may be perceived to be 'secular', from one point of view, may be seen to be value-filled (Franks 2004) or as secularized Christianity (Beckford and

Walliss 2006) from another. A third way that is not binary where the religious is perceived to be 'in the very fabric of the secular' has been proposed, in which many secular practices can be seen to have their roots in religious traditions (Knott 2005, Beckford and Walliss 2006; Knott and Franks 2007). Hanegraaff also takes the middle way in the sociology of religion's unresolved secularization/re-enchantment argument. He sees secularization as a transformation of religion, rather than as the disappearance of it, making the point that society is not based upon 'science and rationality' any more than pre-Enlightenment Christianity was based upon Christian theology. It is not science but popular *mythologies* of *science* that provide society with its basic collective symbolism. (Hanegraaff 1999: 149).

Through the global market and the intensification of the movement of people around the world, we find ourselves in a situation where we have a wealth of religious traditions in their 'traditonal' and revivalist forms, New Age forms and burgeoning 'spiritualities' and quasi-spiritualities in simultaneous and close juxtaposition. One of the unexpected outcomes of this juxtaposition is not the inevitable and blanket dilution of faith but the reinforcement of traditions through dispute, identity issues and competition for resources for religious activities within particular geographical areas. This latter was a particular issue in our study. Hanegraaff sees this 'deregulation of religions' as being 'one of the hidden ironies of secularisation' (1999: 26). So, he does accept the secularization argument to some degree as he sees signs of the 'reinstitutionalisation' of religion and thinks the growth of religious diversity in the UK has exacerbated this (Hanegraaff 1999: 26).

Further, there has been speculation as to the degree to which any religion can be 'traditional' or reflect the original state of the religion in its pristine condition. Mellor and Shilling (1994) have pointed to the notion that all religions are reflexive but that some are more reflexive than others. Reflexivity could be noted in our study, for instance in the differences in Catholicism as practised by the Polish and Dominican interviewees, since their particular practice of Catholicism is skewed by its encounter with culture, nation, homeland, language and custom.

As mentioned above, personalized spiritualities, forms of faith that are embedded in the secular, suit postmodern lifestyles. 'Disadvantageous' doctrines can be discarded and a pick and mix of new dogma from various identified or unidentified sources, can be acquired. Some of our interviewees had developed their own spiritualities, often as a reaction to their disillusionment through their experiences of formal religious worship, especially in relation to congregations. Occasionally they had developed personal forms of ritual through their physical inability to attend a place of worship. Personal spirituality could be said to be the way in which many women, having a need for something other than scientific rationalism, fight back and claim religion for themselves.

Religion and aging

The majority of the women in this study are of an age where they have been brought up in their respective faiths and have remained constant with them. Our first-generation migrant participants, living as they do in settled communities, are associated with established faiths and tend to regard themselves as 'traditional' in their religious practices. An illustration of this is in our Polish group, in particular, who have their own Polish church, with a Polish club and a Polish school, which they have built alongside. They have claimed their own physical, social and religious space, described by one of our participants as 'a little piece of Poland'. The Polish participants, as described in chapter 4, had either been taken as teenagers to the USSR or to Germany as forced labour and the land they inhabited as children has in some cases long ceased to be Poland. It is also the case that British forms of Christianity and Western European secularist lifestyles, frequently influenced by Protestant values, are equally distinctive and related to identity but, because of the hegemony of that value system in the British context, they tend to go unnoticed. Some of the mainly non-migrant participants who are non-practising were reluctant to say for sure that they did not believe in a god or that they know for certain that there is no afterlife. This may be a result of their upbringing and inculcation into religious beliefs and practices 60 or more years ago.

Davie and Vincent (1998) suggest that surveys indicate that the elderly have been more religious than the young. It may be that this statement needs to be geographically and culturally located. Recent research with the African refugee community in a northern English city – dispersed to that city within the last five years – suggests that all participants, children and adults were active in their faith, both Muslims and Christians (Franks 2006). The majority of the literature on faith and aging is written about the experience of American white or African-American Christians, long-term settled communities, and does not explore the effect of changing demographics through migration.

This general lack of a literature is an important gap because, as Davie and Vincent (1998) suggest, the way in which we understand age itself is largely determined by religious understanding of life. For instance, Ram-Prasad (1995) examines the classical Indian idea of treating old age as the last of four stages of life and as a time of renunciation, a time to pass over property and responsibility to the next generation and concentrate on preparing for the next life. He examines this concept, from both a world-embracing and a world-transcending standpoint, and suggests that old age is more significant from the world-transcending (in this case Hindu) point of view. It can be difficult to make sense of aging from a totally secular and world-embracing perspective as from this viewpoint old age might be perceived as a time of loss.

Our group of older women have been largely devout. The majority of our minority ethnic participants told us that they have been devout all their lives and that their religiosity has neither decreased nor increased with age. Only four minority ethnic participants said the importance of their faith had decreased. One of these was an Indian participant, who was now housebound and no longer able to attend the temple that had no lift. One was a Polish Catholic who had been a successful businesswoman and who was now bereaved. Another was a Hindu participant, who had a middle-class lifestyle and the last was a black Caribbean participant who originated from Trinidad. The latter of these, a Catholic, added that even though she no longer attended Mass 'I still say my Hail Mary's'. This was representative of the kind of 'non-practitioner' who has not given up on religious practices altogether. They may still use the symbolism and practice in a way that suited them in communing with 'the meta-empirical framework of meaning' (Hanegraaff 1999).

The degree of religious involvement we found might relate to the fact that the older people's centres, for instance in the Hindu community, tend to be physically associated with temples and devotion is carried on as part of everyday day-centre life. This is, however, not the whole story because the Muslim women, whose centres were not associated with the Mosque, were also devout. Likewise, the black Caribbean participants attend centres not directly associated with places of worship but are themselves mainly devout Catholics and Protestants. The majority of the Polish interviewees said how important their Polish church is to them and they are regular attendees at Mass and reciters of the rosary. Mass is brought into their centre, based as it is near the Polish church. Only one Polish participant out of twenty-seven expressed any doubts about her faith. The 11 white non-migrant 'rural' and semi-rural women interviewed were also mostly church-goers. Two of them expressed doubts but another said that her faith was *the* most important aspect of her quality of life and two semi-rural interviewees also cited their faith as central to their lives. This is not to say that they do not have issues about some of their Church of England congregations' views. One, a divorcee, related how, at a recent discussion about divorce and remarriage, that she thought, 'My giddy aunt. Some people here really are not liberal at all in their views'. Most of the nine white rural and semi-rural church attendees associated a social dimension to their church, finding community, being contected with others and important social space for friendships, overlapping with the physical and spiritual spaces of the church (Eldred 2002).

Faith and identity

Faith for many of our participants is associated with identity. This is clearly the case for the migrant women in relation to their diasporic identities. For diasporic communities religion may be firmly linked with identity, a way of carving an ethnic identity space (Chivallon 2001, cited in Knott 2005), creating a living link between a lost past and the present. There may also be issues of black identity in relation to Pentecostal religion, as MacRobert (1988) and Toulis (1997) have pointed out, as well as an empowerment of women through Pentecostal worship giving women a voice (McClintock Fulkerson 1996).

Interestingly, most of the black Caribbean participants are Catholic, Methodist or Church of England but some also attended black Pentecostal services on occasion. Only one participant said that she was Apostolic Pentecostalist by denomination. There was a degree of flexibility, for instance, in the Dominican participants' Catholicism. A number made their own decisions regarding church attendance, as compared to the generally constant weekly observance of Polish Catholics. This is not to say that some did not attend every day. One of the black Caribbean participants was a member of the Church of Jesus Christ and the Latter Day Saints that, traditionally, has not attracted a great number of black followers. Interviewees have suggested that their faith has helped them through times of severe hardship. This includes their experiences of forced labour in Siberia or Germany for the Polish women as teenagers and the accounts of deep racism experienced by the black Caribbean women in the workplace, for instance (see Chapter 4).

Morris (1991) points out that in surveys church attendance is often used as an indicator of religiosity. The problem with this is not only that it is Christocentric but it also fails to take into account the flexibility that some of our participants have shown in terms of the practice of their faith. This flexibility involves forms of practice that fit with 'believing without belonging' and also 'believing and partially belonging' as in the case of some of our white interviewees, who may have active spiritual lives but who are not regular church attenders or even those who still belong but have ceased to believe. Ainlay et al. (1992) point out that church attendance may decrease not only with spiritual discomfort but also with decreasing mobility. This proved to be the case for some of our participants. To this end interviewees were asked whether they prayed at home and the majority of believers in our study do, whether they attend church, mosque or temple or observe their religious duties at home.

As suggested above, the meaning and value placed on later life is embedded in beliefs, traditions and location. The very shape of the life course varies across belief systems, ethnicity, culture, gender, locality and so on. In lived experience, these aspects are not separate strands. For some the lifeshape is clearly more cyclical, as Ram-Prasad (1995) suggests in his classical Indian view of later life, which is also in four distinct stages. Lawless (1991), following her interviews with white female Pentecostal preachers in the USA, suggested that the shape of the life course is gendered and was more appropriately expressed in terms of blocks by her female participants (Franks 2001b). Further, the way in which participants regard the future and live in the present is coloured by their faith and the way in which the 'next life' is constructed (Knott 1998). Some of the minority ethnic participants told us how they live their lives now in anticipation of the fulfilment of their hopes for the next life. However, no white non-migrant participant spoke in this respect. The trajectory of the life course as linear may be a peculiarly 'Western' and masculine hegemonic formulation. Viewed from a viewpoint of spatiality, a trajectory has a definite beginning and clear end. It is singular and focused, with the notion of travelling at full speed also being evoked, whereas from more spiritual and cultural viewpoints life cycles and rebirth or a continuation of life evoke the contours and rhythms of life rather than trajectories.

Reflexivity and spiritualities

A response to our data might be that there are two kinds of believer: 'traditional' and 'reflexive'. However, this would be to make something of a false dichotomy because all religious traditions are reflexive to some degree (Mellor 1993). Yet, some traditions are more reflexive than others (Mellor 1993). This reflexive spirit is, for Mellor and Shilling, linked to the 'Protestant template' of 'individualization and the thirst for knowledge' (Mellor and Shilling 1994: 35). It also relates to choice, something which many of the first generation migrant women we have interviewed may not have had regarding their religious affiliations. Because of their age the majority of our participants have started out as believers in their respective faiths and in general it is the Christians, especially the white English Christians, who have been the most apparently reflexive. This is perhaps because they have been most subjected to individualizing, personalizing and secularizing influences, experiences and education in a liberal, secularized Christian environ-ment. Racism and lack of educational opportunities, for instance to learn English, mean that many of the minority ethnic women have been secluded within their own communities. Nevertheless, there were also examples of minority ethnic women being equally reflexive, for instance in responding creatively to lack of mobility or transport by creating their prayer 'spaces' within their homes. A Dominican parti-cipant, a grandmother of 21 grandchildren and 21 great-grandchildren, who depended on her children to transport her to Mass, resorted to buying her own candles and praying at home:

Well I go to Mass when the children take me but in my house I buy candles by the hundred. Every blessed night I light a candle and (when) I say my prayers and I pray to God and I pray, I don't pray for myself alone.

Another black Caribbean woman aged 60, who also came from the Windward Island of Dominica, some 40 years ago, is not a church-goer. Like some of the white non-migrant participants she is critical of church congregations:

I was never really a church person. Never. Um, sometimes I see the people that go to church and, er, they seem to do such awful things. I don't know, probably the little faith I had seemed to diminish.

She also describes a form of spirituality that she has developed in dialogue with her life and environment. She describes a morality that is linked to a meta-empirical framework of justice and involves treating people as she would expect to be treated herself.

Apart from exhibiting reflexivity, this could constitute a case of 'believing but not belonging'. This is interesting in terms of the association of 'New Age' beliefs with the white ethnic majority, because it shows such beliefs to be not exclusive to the white middle or aspiring middle classes (Sutcliffe 2003). Such a belief may be considered as 'popular religion' but it also chimes with the concept of *karma* (the sum of people's actions in previous states of existence, viewed as deciding their fate in future ones) in the Hindu religion.

Among 'traditional religions' there is structural reflexivity, which takes place through the encounter of religions and belief systems in a geographical context. All first-generation migrants will have been subject to these changes. For instance, the participant cited below relates how the encounter with racism and social exclusion, resulting from migration, intensified the religiosity of first-generation black Caribbean migrants. She said:

I came here in 1962 and thing's wasn't beautiful ... but at least we got over the hatred. And we tried to forgive and tried to live because we put God in front of us we ... we were Christians before we came here but, we go deeper into Christianity here, more than home. Because the things that we met when we come to here, we didn't have at home. The abuse and the neglect, you know? Even in work.

Ballard has pointed out how Indian religions have become more separate in the UK through the process of migration but that Punjabi religion, for instance, still incorporates Hindus and Sikhs (Kalsi 1992; Chohan 2001; Ballard 2000). The Punjabi ethnic and cultural ties take precedence over religious difference. This was evident at a focus group held at a Hindu temple where both Hindu and Sikh older women meet. A Sikh participant illustrated the point by saying, 'I would go to a Mosque if I was invited'.

As mentioned previously, the reflexivity among the migrant and non-migrant Christian participants and the development of a personal kind of spirituality seems to relate to disillusion with the behaviour of others in the context of the church. A rural participant, quoted earlier, expressed a natural theology developed through the observation of nature:

> I seem to think there is something there. When I look at things in life, I think things are so marvellous, how everything works and life, you know, it is so complicated and, yet, everything fits in, all the different animals they all have their different purposes. I feel there is something, you know, but I don't just know how to explain it.

Reflexivity also relates to having the opportunity to move freely in public social spaces, beyond the immediate home and community (which implies ability to speak the dominant language), as well as having access to information. It is not easy for older women to commune with nature or the environment, for example, from inner city locations. There is also, therefore, an issue about lack of opportunity to access the rural (Dhalech 1999).

One Polish interviewee had found herself doubting since the death of her husband, and she had grown to have a kind of questioning faith, which seemed more general among some of the white non-migrant respondents. She said:

> Well the truth is I still believe in my religion. I think I am much wiser now than when I was young. When I was young, I did everything my parents said and we listen[ed] to our church – what our church said. But now when I have travelled all over the world ... and I have seen different religions and sometimes it makes me think 'is there really a God?' I can't really say because I am frightened to say if it is true or not.

There were also the more affluent white women who talked about the importance of prayer and who were equally as devout as the majority of the minority ethnic women. In the main the faith of the Christian black Caribbean and white non-migrant women tended to be more reflexive and they did not experience their doubt as irreconcilable with belief. The vast majority of South Asian participants expressed no doubt at all. Those white contributors, who had moved to another part of the country in retirement, had more frequently developed personal forms of spirituality. There is evidence of kinds of spirituality, which are neither defined by the participants as 'religion' but nor are they rationalist beliefs. For this reason they fit more comfortably with the notion of 'popular or vernacular religion' (Sutcliffe 2003).

Social benefits

The benefits of attendance at worship and being part of a faith community were reported as being many and include social benefits. This is not to say that our participants associate themselves with places of worship for social benefit alone, but in practice it is difficult to separate out the social from these other benefits as they intersect. The social significance of communal worship is especially the case for widows and single women. The only never-married women we encountered were among the white more affluent participants. It is a fact that places of worship (apart from the mosque) are among the few places where older women can comfortably go alone, make friends and be part of a community. The Muslim women had other arrangements, holding gatherings in their homes. Such assemblies include reading groups and prayer meetings, remembering the dead, such as the gathering a widowed participant held in memory of her husband. During the fieldwork process of a subsequent research project, a Pakistani interviewer found that an easy place to meet women was at the *Janazah*, when paying respects for the dead, where women sit together for a few hours and get talking (Afshar et al. 2006).

A Muslim widow in our older women research told us that she attended a special meeting every Thursday for two hours of silent prayer. Some Muslim women who were widows found themselves isolated and depressed and one women's group in particular had been founded to combat this isolation. One Muslim participant told us that she was used to her isolation and that her faith helps her to cope with it. When she feels depressed, she engages in religious activity.

The social benefits to women who live alone were expressed by a black Caribbean contributor as:

> It helps a lot 'cause they're always there for you. Somebody always comes to see you especially if you live alone.

A white never-married contributor recounts how:

> Moving into a place on your own, as I did, and I'd been thirty years in my old parish in Sussex and I went to church and I thought 'I'm not leaving this church until I've spoken to somebody'. And I went up to X and I said 'Hello, I'm new to the parish' and he then introduced me to Y ... and then Z wanted people to help with the jumble sale at the church. Well, I was in then.

Some places of worship offered the opportunity to get involved in a range of activities. As a white rural participant described:

> Well they have this three Saturdays in the year they have Dickensian Saturdays here at the church house. We do coffee and mince pies three Saturdays and we take thousands of pounds actually because visitors come from all over and we dress up in Victorian costume.

There are opportunities to read aloud from scripture and to 'help out' at temple or church. The latter often involves domestic tasks, such as tea-making and tea- and cake-selling (churches) or food preparation, laundry or getting ready lights for worship (temples). These activities bring contact with others, as well as setting tasks, thereby offering a sense of functionality. A Gujarati Hindu contributor demonstrated how she would make purified ghee candles that are used for *Aarti* at the Mandir – different kinds of candles for different Gods. She explained via an interpreter how she would wash the clothes and the tea towels and clean the copper things. A 69-year-old Sikh respondent, who goes to the Gurdwara two or three days a week, makes a useful contribution and confirms herself as part of a community that is wider than family and friends alone. This sense of connectedness and belonging has also been suggested by Eldred (2002) in relation to older white Christian women, as part of church community life for older white women.

Some participants have friendship networks, which are formed at the church but which also function outside of that setting, becoming part of everyday life and an ongoing support system. As discussed in Chapter 5, for white internal migrants *within* the UK, this can become a way of reconstructing kin. For one of the latter, however, a principle had to be put before the social benefits that her church bestowed upon her. This contributor, aged 70 and never married, had developed close friendships and a social life based around her Anglican Church. She had taken up the study of theology in her retirement and went on to do theological research for a PhD. However, her changing theology meant that she decided she had to forgo this safe environment because she could not ignore the fact that the vicar was opposed to the ordination of women. She wrote and explained this to the vicar and to her friends. She now attends another church, where she has yet to develop friendships. The old friendships continue but they see each other less often. Her friends found it difficult to understand why she would take this principled step at the cost of the social benefits and thought it would have been better to have kept quiet. This implies the possibility of 'belonging and not believing' mentioned earlier.

Prayer

There are similarities between the minority ethnic participants in terms of their general unwavering devoutness and their belief in the efficacy of prayer. Many had a sense of being watched over by divine powers, which gave little room for doubt. Prayer was deeply important to the majority of participants who were believers from all faiths. A sense of peace through prayer was mentioned by some, as well as the encouragement to be a better person and to get along better with others. Being close to Allah and feeling clean, even the importance of prayer (*salat*) as a form of physical exercise was mentioned by some Muslim participants. For the Hindus prayer was important as constant remembrance and singing *bhajans* (sacred chants) was a favourite pastime for a number of Hindu participants. They do *puja* (make offerings) in their homes, where all have a little shrine, but they also attend *Aarti* at the Mandir or Hindu Community Centre and then continue to sing *bhajans* and pray at their day centres. They call on the gods before embarking on an enterprise and in times of need. Some women reported how they had more time to pray now that they were older. For instance, a Polish interviewee said 'When I was working, I was too busy and too occupied so I only Sunday got to church but during the week I didn't have much time to pray'. But now, along with others in our study, she spends a great deal more time in prayer.

There were Christian migrant women who also reported having their prayers answered, sometimes in a spectacular way. For instance, a Dominican grandmother of 27 grandchildren and 14 'great grans', recounted how she was suffering from a form of glaucoma and regained her sight after, in her desperation, she shouted at God from her hospital bed. She told us how in the morning her son came to visit and she realized that she could see. A Polish woman, who was sent to forced labour in Germany at the age of 15 and made to dig trenches on the front line, came to England at the close of the Second World War and was sent to work in a mill. Traumatized by the low-flying bombers that made the earth shake, she was deeply frightened of the noise level in the weaving-room. Fortunately she was sent to learn burling and mending (a highly skilled invisible mending technique) but acquiring the skill through imitation and, without the English language, was defeating her. Desperately unhappy she prayed to the Virgin Mary as she had done every night since she had been taken from her home. She related how that night in a dream, she was instructed exactly how to perform the task on the three large holes in fabric on which she was learning. In her dream she followed the instructions, starting with the easiest and working towards the most difficult hole. The next day she worked just as she had done in the dream. She said:

> [W]hen I got up in the morning I got to work and I sat there and I thought 'Wait a minute. How did I do it? I started it so and so and so. And I started it just the way I dreamt it and, you know, from that day I never had any difficulty.

One black Caribbean Methodist respondent described how she had lost her handbag in New York City. This meant that she had no passport and she fasted and prayed because she wanted to be permitted to go home. When she returned to the UK, a woman who had found the handbag in the New York taxi where it had been left returned it to her. Of the power of prayer she said:

> I can talk to God like how I'm talking to you, I don't see Him but I can talk to Him because if I have a problem or if I have the arthritis in me

knee I can say 'do God and ease these two knees, these two legs not only for myself but for other people'. An' sometimes, you know, it's not better but you can get a little upliftment from it an' so that's why when I'm, uh, inside I don't have that big loneliness because I know God is there, you know.

Among the Hindus there were also those who attributed improvement in health and well-being to prayer. One said, for instance, that through prayer 'the body will stay nice and even feel better, as well, and your health ... not completely but health-wise it makes you want to go and do more things'. Concerns over money could also be the subject of prayer. Two Hindu participants told how they could pray to Lakshmi if they were in need of money and a black Caribbean Catholic related how, if she prayed when she was in need of money, help always came from somewhere.

Some respondents had been helped in bereavement, not only in terms of a sense of support and intimacy but in feeling they were able to communicate in some way with their loved-ones, as is discussed in the next chapter. There was also the possibility to forgive in the face of overt racism in the workplace as was expressed in discussion with a black Caribbean focus group. The power and capacity to forgive in a situation where there is still a reluctance to talk about the past to strangers because 'our grief would fill this room' was electrifying.

Others participants spoke of the emotional support they gained from their faith, which they said helped them to cope with their day-to-day difficulties. A Muslim participant, whose husband suffered from mental illness and who had not been able to speak to her for many years, said that her 'religion has influenced my life very positively and this has helped me to care for my husband and help cope with stressful events'. Other Muslims commented on how they gained a sense of peace from their prayers and had been helped in bereavement. Women from different faiths, who had acted as long-term carers of their husbands, appeared to have gained comfort from their faith even after their death . Another Muslim participant commented, 'I pray five times a day, this helps me to deal with family traumas and upsets'.

Prayer is important to all the devout women, with the pattern of prayer of different kinds woven into the fabric of their lives. The majority of the older Hindu women sing *bhajans* and said that this was one of their favourite pastimes along with (for those who could read Gujarati) reading holy texts in their own language. One Hindu woman, who lives on her own wakes up at 6 a.m. and prays, reads from her Gujarati book and sings hymns every morning. This reading of holy texts was also important to the Muslim women, while some of the black Caribbean women also spent time reading the Bible or attending Bible classes. Some of the white women also engage in these activities.

Pilgrimage

Temples and churches organize trips abroad, which are frequently linked to pilgrimage. Pilgrimages offer not only a spiritual dimension but an opportunity for women to travel unaccompanied as part of the pilgrim group. Several women had been on a number of pilgrimages to the holy places of their respective faiths and this was especially the case for the Muslims, the Hindus and the Polish participants, who had been to Mecca in Saudi Arabia, to India, and to Europe to visit Rome, Lourdes and Fatima, respectively. Some Muslim participants who had not made pilgrimages had hopes for the future, which included saving enough money to go on the Hajj and praying that they would be able to travel to Mecca. Some of the older Muslim women had already been on the Hajj on more than one occasion, although the Muslim requirement regarding Hajj as a pillar of Islam is to carry out the pilgrimage once in a lifetime. One, for example, had been six times. Muslim participants who had been on the *Hajj*, one of the Five Pillars of Islam, said that they gained in respect within their families and communities as a result, but were anxious to make the point to us that this was not their reason for going.

Pilgrimage is distinct from 'holidaymaking'. It is a spiritual undertaking, but nevertheless involves making a physical journey that for some participants clearly had a social side. A Polish interviewee, a widow, explained how she liked to go to Lourdes and Fatima and that she had been to Israel three times, as well as to Rome 'to see the Pope' and to Assisi. When asked what she had got out of it she replied:

Goodness. Much goodness. Much nice people and, um, I feel much better each time I went. I was always travelling nearly every year somewhere.

For some Hindus, Mother India, India in itself, is a Goddess, a holy place and the Ganges too is a god. During a research visit to a Hindu temple as part of our study, Hindus were taking their leave of the community centre and were presented with flowers and coconuts. They were setting off to India and the researcher was informed that coconuts are a symbolic sacrifice from the community to throw into the River Ganges as a means of atonement. The white Christian theologian mentioned earlier also saw the significance for herself in pilgrimage. For her the study of theology was itself a form of pilgrimage, a spiritual and intellectual journey, albeit it in a mental landscape. For a woman living alone this was a journey not without its dangers, in that her changing understanding of her faith meant that she had also had to change her place of worship and marginalize herself to some degree from old friends.

Doubt and individual spiritual beliefs

The more personalized spiritual beliefs were generally expressed by members of the white more affluent group. Personal beliefs included ideas such as meeting everyone you have ever known on one's death, feeling that there must be someone watching over you or that somehow we all get our just desserts, the latter being associated with a sense of an overarching justice. As mentioned above, this shift from traditional faith seems to have taken place in the white non-migrant population more than it has in that of the minority ethnic contributors. This may have something to do with age, as well as to exposure to mainstream culture, as the participants involved are all at the younger end of the age range of those in the study. All have been in full-time employment and have been exposed through music, the media and sometimes personal experience to New Age and spiritual ideas, often an eclectic formation from a mixture of religions that has become especially prevalent since the 1960s.

There were also those involved in non-religious groups based upon ethical concerns, such as the rural participant who is involved in the peace movement. Although this respondent attended church, she expressed some disillusion and doubt concerning the Christian faith and in particular its practices, for instance, her church investing in War Bonds. She made courageous contributions to, and gained a sense of moral fulfilment from, her exertions for the peace movement. At times she had risked arrest on account of her work in this respect:

> And I also went to Molesworth on a demonstration. And that was quite moving because some of the peace demonstrators had built a little church out of twigs. I saw somebody being arrested, X. The police linked arms like this and I wouldn't have believed it if I hadn't seen it. They linked arms and they charged into the crowd and they arrested X from Y hospital so he couldn't go home on the coach. And I've also been with Mothers for Peace to Russia.

Exclusion and curtailment of religious participation

Ainlay et al. (1992) found that health has a mediating role in church participation and it was evident that, with increasing age and decreased mobility, some participants found themselves excluded from what had been the mainstay of their lives up until this point. Some of the more disabled Polish women are bussed to the Polish Church on a Sunday by community transport and the priest takes Mass and Confession to their community centre, located as it is only a couple of buildings along the street from the church. Church of England services were also taken to a sheltered housing group of mainly white inner-city women. One white working-class woman who is 80 and a Methodist said, 'I used to go (to church) a lot but now I can't get up. I can't sit long'. The church now takes Holy Communion to her and she says that religion has helped her to get through her illnesses. The problem associated with attendance at the temple was, according to a Hindu community leader, particularly one for older Hindu women who are in living in residential homes where non-Hindu workers do not recognize the significance of such attendance. There was also an issue for a housebound participant who could not manage the temple stairs.

Although the issue of exclusion is often in terms of access to public worship, there is also for the less able-bodied a problem of exclusion from the possibility of private worship too. This is an important part of the daily routine for many of the devout participants, for instance the Hindus who make *puja* morning and evening and make their offerings before they eat, the Sikhs who do not breakfast until they have prayed, and the Muslims who also rise early and pray five times a day. One

Muslim participant who is 63 explained how religion is her main interest and she used to spend time reading religious books. However, her eyesight is now too bad. A Hindu woman and our oldest interviewee in her 80s was totally excluded, both from the local day centre and the *mandir*, through the lack of a lift (a grant had been unsuccessfully applied for). She and another participant were no longer able to do *puja* at home because their hands shake when they hold a candle. She, therefore, has to limit herself to reciting the names of the gods and goddesses.

Nevertheless, exclusion through lack of mobility does not necessarily stop our participants from practising their faith. For instance, we have already seen how one black Caribbean participant cannot get to Mass unless taken, so she prays at home and lights her own candles for the purpose. She did not let her absence from church stop her from living out her social gospel. She gave an inspiring account of her activities on the part of a Dominican young man whom she saw in the street looking 'like a tramp' and who had recently come out of prison. She took him to her house, 'a big man', made him bath, cut his hair, told him to sleep on the sofa, sent him to the benefits office the next day, helped him find a flat, and gave him pots and pans and sheets. She said that she did this because she believes in helping people. The literature suggests it may also be because of her cultural status as a black Caribbean grandmother that she would show such generosity to this young man (Plaza 2000; Pulsipher 1993). This participant is powerful at the same time as she is 'depowered'. She is old, has angina, was hospitalized for thrombosis and still experiences pain in her leg. She has been blind in one eye from birth. She gave birth to ten children, three of whom died. Yet she negotiates and mediates with families in her neighbourhood in an attempt to 'bring peace to their homes'. She squares up to men and informs them of their duty. She is powerful in a way that older women in British society are somehow not expected to be.

The older, less able-bodied Pakistani Muslim women, some of whom live alone, pray standing up. A white non-migrant participant talked about how she and her husband no longer attend church, as he is now unable to sit for extended periods of time and, therefore, her role as carer kept her away from church. Other participants have to take taxis to Mass on Sundays because there is no Sunday bus. A Hindu interviewee said that she could only go to the temple, a short distance away, in daylight.

Some of our Muslim participants had been asked to act as consultants by the local council and had informed them about Muslim hygiene requirements, as well as the need for prayer mats and prayer space in residential settings. There is a need for the provision of faith-sensitive services if people are not to be excluded from mainstream health-care provision and other forms of support, for reasons of their religious practices. Gilliat-Ray has pointed out how inappropriate services may be thrust on people if their religious requirements are simply understood by rote. She gives the example of Muslims in a hospital forced to face Mecca at all times, even though they would only face Mecca to pray and they may, in fact, not have been practising Muslims at all (Gilliat-Ray 2001). A Muslim participant who is a widow aged 64 told us that she will not go to hospital for the treatment she badly needs because she will miss her ritual prayers.

It has been seen that many of our participants were dependent on relatives to take them to worship. These findings are in keeping with those of Koenig et al. (1988) who found that although devotion increased with age, attendance at worship decreased. Ainlay et al. (1992) have suggested that such a decrease is due to disability. However, the opportunities for and limitations to private worship need to be factored into this equation, as well as their effects on older people's faith and sense of well-being.

Conclusion

At a time when faith is popularly seen as becoming less socially important but at the same time is being put on the agenda in terms of diversity management, it has to be said that for the older women in this study a lack of faith was something of an exception rather than a rule, especially among the minority ethnic women. Many of the white women also spoke about their faith and rejection of church-going frequently manifested itself alongside personal spiritualities. At times this was a partial rejection, a 'believing and partially belonging'. What these participants frequently rejected was the institution and the social behaviour within the setting of the church. Only one of these white participants claimed outright that she did not have some spiritual belief and the interviews and focus group discussions offer insight into the intensity of many of the participants' views. Black (1999) has recorded the narratives of older poor African-American women in the USA and how their spirituality is a means of their empowerment. For some of our participants their faith is the very meaning of their existence, 'second only to our lives', as one black Caribbean participant expressed it. Religion does not come alone and it cannot be separated out from issues of identity, ethnicity and culture. Fundamentalists attempt to isolate religion and say that it is possible to practise it in a vacuum, divorced from culture. But here we were presented with the living network of women's lives in which the religious strand is woven into the fabric and connected to all the other aspects of this. It is an integer in their quality of life. Stephen Sapp (1987) writes that much of the Christian writing on old age is over-optimistic, painting it with a rose tint and avoiding the reality of suffering, but he criticizes a value system that measures the worth of people by what they do. Religion is not here being recommended as a panacea for later life but merely as an aspect of quality of life that needs to be taken into account in any analysis of aging.

The impact of religion should not be ignored in making an analysis of issues of empowerment and disempowerment in older women's lives. We have already seen in Chapter 3 that our participants from a post-gerontological viewpoint are simultaneously empowered and disempowered in other ways. Empowerment is not binary and nor is belief. Spirituality and religion are neither all empowering nor totally disempowering. It could be argued that religion has disempowered many of our women in specific ways, for instance through isolating them from the wider community. But their isolation also stems from culture, ethnicity, racism, lack of mobility, lack of opportunity to learn English and so on. They have called upon their faith to sustain them through the difficulties. It is important then that religious aspects be taken into account in planning and policy-making when considering the current elderly generation. At times they may find themselves excluded from mainstream services due to a plethora of causes, one of which may be a lack of sensitivity on the part of providers to issues of faith.

8

Death, dying and widowhood

Introduction

Death is largely seen as the province of the elderly and, therefore, normalized; it tends to be taken for granted and treated in a common-sense kind of way. In Western cultures there is a tendency to see death as 'timely' or 'untimely' (Sidell 1994). Whereas dying at a young age is regarded as tragic or premature, the death of an older person evokes phrases such as having 'had a good innings' or 'lived to a ripe old age'. Most deaths in Western societies occur at older ages. Further, the ability to prolong life, due to advancement in medicine and technology, means that death itself has become something of a medical event and its occurrence may be regarded as a medical failure (Seale 1998; Debate of the Age Health and Care Study Group 1999; Howarth 2006). Most Britons die in hospital, even though they say they would prefer to die at home (Smith 2000). As Smith says, today, a 'soulless death in intensive care is the most modern of deaths' (2000: 129).

Not withstanding this, death is something of a taboo subject in the West. Both as individuals and collectively, we tend to be wary of death, exhibiting discomfort and embarrassment in the face of it. We find it difficult to come to terms with those who are dying and often go out of our way to avoid people who have been bereaved (Seale 1998). Gorer (1965), for example, has written that sex has been replaced by death as the main taboo subject in contemporary society and that we have become death-denying. Moreover, while there has been a proliferation of writing on the topic in recent years, this has mainly focused on palliative care and the idea of encouraging service providers to facilitate a 'good death' (Smith 2000; Carr 2003). There is a dearth of studies on older people's own views of death and dying, even though there is some evidence that older people think about it and are prepared to discuss it calmly and without anxiety (Carr 2003; Coleman 1994; Hallberg 2004). Indeed, this proved to be the case with the participants in this study, most of whom have lost loved ones and some of whom have had brushes with death themselves. Further, the variables of gender, ethnicity and faith community in relation to these views comprise rich territories that are waiting to be explored (Field et al. 1997).

This chapter is organized in five further sections. The first of these examines what is known about societal attitudes to death and dying. It explores these issues in relation to death as a taboo subject and in terms of claims about the secularization of death. The second section examines women's experiences of bereavement, which has occurred across the life course. It then looks at our participants' feelings about their own death. Here it is found that most accept it as fact and are more than willing to talk about it. While they do not fear death *per se*, most are concerned about what will lead up to departure, especially in relation to pain, notions of dignity and worries about burdening family. The fourth section looks at our women's experiences of widowhood. As a form of bereavement, this is treated in a category of its own as it is a time replete with pain, unconscionable grief and trauma. The final section draws the chapter together by making some concluding remarks.

Attitudes to death and dying

According to writers such as Aries (1983) and Elias (1985), in Western societies, prior to the 20th century, dying took place in the presence of others, especially friends and relations and sometimes other members of the community. However, death gradually came to be characterized by silence and denial. It was kept hidden by talking instead about illness, thereby implying a cure by putting those who were dying in hospital, away from public view, and by the medicalization of death by the medical profession for whom it represents failure. As Aries says, 'we have removed death from society, eliminated its character of public

141

ceremony, and made it a private act' (1983: 575). For Elias, 'never before in the history of humanity have the dying been removed so hygienically behind the scenes of social life' (1985: 23).

However, while there is much to suggest that death is a relatively hidden event and a prohibited topic, there are differing perspectives on this. Armstrong (1987), for instance, argues that it is not so much that there is silence about death but a new way of speaking about it and a preoccupation with the dead body. This is because of the legal requirement that the cause of death must be medically certified and the significance of the fact that the first thing that occurs after a death is that a doctor is summoned. Walter (1994) questions how far the denial of death is, in fact, a modern phenomenon, indicating instead that it is part of the human condition in which fear of dying is universal. He suggests that it is not society as whole that denies death currently but certain professional groups. This is particularly so for the medical profession and for those working in the mass media with their preoccupation with youth and glamour. Wouters (2002) points out, however, that in most Western countries, particularly northern Europe and North America, there have been recent changes in thinking about and confronting death. Those who are dying are now usually told about this and are able to go through a form of 'anticipatory mourning', alongside those who are closest to them. Although in the 1960s and 1970s mourning became increasingly privatized and individualized, there has recently been a move for new kinds of rituals to be sought. Mourning is, therefore, both a highly institutionalized social obligation and a very individualized and personal process. It, thus, includes both public and private actions and feelings.

Yet the arguments discussed above are not in themselves unproblematic. For it needs to be pointed out that they are very Westernized and ethnocentric. They are rooted in assumptions about Christianity and associated notions of secularization, which may not hold for minority ethnic cultures and their religious beliefs and practices or indeed for other groups. For instance, it is often suggested that there has been a decline in the influence of religion to the extent that death has lost its meaning and is no longer seen as part of a divine plan or as a step from life to the afterlife. Due to the processes of secularization, death itself has been secularized (Walter 1996; Brown 2001). Yet these discussions are concerned with Christianity alone. Further, there is disagreement as to the extent to which such secularization might be said to have occurred. Walter (1996), for example, argues that although the Christian religions may have declined in an institutional sense, as evinced in decreased attendance at places of formal worship, this does not mean that people do not adhere to certain kinds of religious belief. These are simply hidden, rather than more apparent. Beliefs about death and what comes after have become 'personally meaningful but socially irrelevant' (Walter 1996: 192).

This is supported by the fact that significant numbers of those living in the UK consistently report that they have a religious affinity. The 2001 Census, for instance, indicated that just over three-quarters of the British population reported having a religion, with 72 percent citing Christianity and nearly 3 percent Islam (National Statistics 2004). The next largest religious groups were Hindus, Sikhs, Jews and Buddhists, respectively. Further, although the religious question was a voluntary one in the Census, over 92 percent of people chose to answer it. Indeed, as reported in the previous chapter, a very high proportion of the participants in our study put claim to having some kind of faith. Such faith is clearly important in influencing individuals' views about death and what happens after it. Many minority ethnic faiths see it as an opening to a worthwhile future (Levin 1994).

For instance, for Muslims, death is to be accepted because it is the will of Allah and Allah establishes its time and circumstances. This world is regarded as a mere passage towards a better future elsewhere. Life is seen as a time of probation and a person will be faced with all their words and deeds at the final judgement. As death approaches, relatives and members of the local community gather round the dying person, making peace with them, praying and citing verses from the Qur'an. After death, rituals concerning how the body is treated need to be observed.

For Hindus and Sikhs, reincarnation has a particular influence on how death is viewed. Time is cyclical, a round of birth, death and rebirth. Any particular life is only one of a cycle. Hindus, for example, believe that the true aim of life is to free the soul to be with the god, Krishna. A soul reincarnates again and again on earth until it becomes perfect and the state of godliness is reached. Moreover, whether a soul is reborn in a human or non-human form depends on its moral state. That which is sewn in one lifetime will be reaped in another. A dying

Hindu should have their family gathered round them and should die with the name of Krishna being recited.

Similarly, for Sikhs, human life is just a stage in the upward march of the soul. An individual human being is born after going through lower forms of life. Humanity is the soul's final stage in the progression to divinity. Sikhism believes in the immortality of the soul. After death a Sikh faces the next birth according to how the previous life has been lived. If a person has committed evil, they are reborn as a lower species and the reincarnation cycle begins again. If they have behaved well, then they will be reborn into a better life. The only way out of this cycle of reincarnation is to achieve total knowledge and union with God. Along with other religions, believers who are dying should ideally be surrounded by family and friends. These will recite from the Holy book and death should take place with the name of God being recited.

Although many of the religious customs of minority ethnic groups have been adapted to suit life in the UK, it is clear from what follows below that faith and spirituality remain important in our participants' views about death, dying and bereavement. There are also likely to be degrees of flexibility in the ways in which people apply and interpret their religious principles, as the discussion in the previous chapter has also shown. The women whom we interviewed were, by the simple fact of their age bracket, living in the shadow of death and many were aware of this fact. Some were preparing for the departure, some looked forward to it, while others were simply enjoying the current phase of their lives and did not find it necessary to look too far beyond. What our participants demonstrate, however, is that it is not easy to generalize about death and the experience of the death of others.

Experiences of bereavement

As might be expected of women of their age, all our participants had experienced death of one kind or another. Several had lost children and it was agreed that this was a terrible bereavement. One of the African-Caribbean participants, for instance, had lost three out of her ten children. The first died after an accident at the childminders. As a result, although this woman had to work, she vowed never to use a childminder again:

So, from that, I get myself expect another child and I say 'I don't care if I drink salt water, I not going to give my children for baby minder again. And that's why I had to stay at home and look after them.

Widowhood also occasioned terrible pain, sense of loss and mourning, as described later in the chapter. Most of our respondents' parents were also dead, with a few speaking of how this had occurred when they were very young. For instance, a black Caribbean participant aged 76 had lost her parents when she was seven on the small island where she was born. This had left her as head of the household. She told us:

My father died there. My mother died there. And when they die they leave the house and four girls and four boys and my big sister was hurricane killing her. So I am the second.

The extended family came to the rescue and provided her with a home.

Another of our participants, who had lost her parents as a child, had been taken in by people on the Island of Dominica, where she was used to help with housework and do the ironing. However, she had not been allowed to go to school or have an education. Unsurprisingly she felt that this had caused difficulties for her throughout her life. A 60-year-old from the same island spoke of how early childhood experiences had made her fear death in her youth, that she was relieved to have lived long enough to have grown old and that she intended to make the most of the remainder of her life:

My mum died when I was quite young and I prayed that I wouldn't die with my boots on at work. I even threatened them, if I die with my boots on, if I die before I retire, you're in trouble. I'm going to be appearing all the time. [Lots of laughter] And I've retired now and I just want to enjoy my peace. Life is short.

For some of the Polish participants, in particular, who had lost parents and siblings when they were teenagers during the war, there remained deep scars of dark memories that had affected their whole lives. As described in Chapter 4, their stories were indeed harrowing. One told us that when she was 18:

My mother died. My brother, a little boy, died. All the old people and children all died.

As reported earlier in the book, another said:

I was 18. My mother died after three months because all old people and all children die because hungry and cold. We [were] very hungry, very short of food. Terrible. Terrible ... Nine months is snow in Siberia. My mother died 7 May. It was still with snow. And they have to dig in the snow. Dig in the ground because, you know, it was frozen and bury without coffin like a dog. And living in the forest so many would [die] but it was no coffin. Nobody has a coffin.

One Polish commentator described how her family was thrown out of their country and transported to Germany. Her father had died after two months and her mother shortly afterwards. This left her and her three siblings to fend for themselves.

Losing brothers and sisters was also hard to cope with. A Dominican participant, who had lost her sister, felt that only faith had given her the strength to cope:

So she die and I pray to God and God make me able to bear it.

The women also recounted the significance in their lives of having lost other relatives and friends. The death of daughters and brothers-in-law was reported as well as mothers and fathers-in-law. Even when expected, these bereavements tended to have huge implications for the family life. As one white working-class woman put it, the death of her daughter-in-law, 'knocked us for six'. The death of friends was also important, signalling to older women their own mortality. During the interviews, participants produced photographs and mementos of holidays and outings, often indicating that others, who were with them then, had now passed on. One of the middle-class, single, rural women, whose close friend had been killed in a road accident four years previously, said that 'I miss her very, very much ... and we had a lot of fun together'. Another, who was married, had a long-standing best friend who was suffering with cancer and undergoing chemotherapy. She talked about being 'sobered' by the experience and that it had made her reflect more closely on the current stage of her own life and mortality.

The women had also had other experiences in relation to dying. Several had had near brushes with death themselves, as with the African-Caribbean participant who had nearly died during childbirth and had been given the last rites. One of the white working-class women's husbands had nearly died while she was pregnant with her fifth child. He had subsequently never been able to hold down a job and she had to run their off-licence business on her own. Several of the white inner-city women reported early experiences of death as a result of the Second World War, either through the loss of family members or friends or via their own involvement in the war effort. One woman explained, for instance, how she had worked as a cleaner in a sanatorium, which mainly cared for men from the armed forces who had contracted tuberculosis. Commenting on how men who had survived the war then died from the diseases they had contracted, she indicated:

> All of them and a lot died. Yes. We'd go in each morning and 'how's Jimmy doing and how's … oh, he's gone'. You'd see his empty bed.

This contributor, reflecting on the good lives that had been given, wondered whether the war had been worth it. She said:

> all them good lives that they give that were lost for what we have today – has it been worth it? I don't think so. A lot of us don't think so. We're losing all those lives for the lives we've got today – mugging, vandalism, all this. Why did they have to lose their lives? For what?

Two main points arise from the above discussions. The first relates to the significance of death in these older women's lives, since everyone had something to say about the subject in relation to their immediate and extended families. This is not then a topic that is taboo or irrelevant for their generation. It, therefore, follows that when commentators on death and dying suggest that they are a source of social denial, they are doing so from a position that ignores the experiences of older people. As with researchers on other areas of social life, the position they adopt is that of what is perceived to be the majority, those in the younger age groups, rather than the elderly themselves. In this they serve to marginalize older people in a field of experience that is ironically largely their preserve.

Second, our study indicates that for this generation of older women, experiences of death and dying have been encountered throughout the life course. As with other issues in this book, these have impacted significantly on our women's lives throughout this time and still have resonances for them today.

Facing up to death

Their own death was regarded as something to be anticipated by women across the different backgrounds. The following describes some of the accepting and fatalistic sentiments that were expressed. For instance, one 80-year-old Hindu woman said; 'You have to go in the end'. A 64-year-old Pakistani woman said that she only talked to her more elderly friends and didn't want to speak to the younger ones, with their tendency to be morbid:

That's why I am peaceful. I don't want to listen to anybody who is fed up or people who talk about dying. I know I am going to die [laughs]

A 64-year-old African-Caribbean woman explained:

I am grateful for everyday I get up. I have another day of life. For me, it's a bonus and I'm grateful for that and I try to enjoy every day and take each day as it comes.

Similarly, a white working-class woman told us:

Oh just pray that I wake up in the morning [laughs]. We always say when we leave each other in the evening, 'I'll see you in the morning, God willing' [laughs].

Another said:

Everyday when you get up it's a bonus ... it's a bonus. It is when you get to my age, anyway.

The Polish women also expressed similar sentiments. For example, a 72-year-old indicated:

People I know just drop dead, so every week is a funeral, really. So, if I see that, you always ... But you never know the future, really. You can't make any future because you don't know the future, you know. Maybe alright today and tomorrow gone. So can't make a future.

Another who is aged 79 explained how she wanted to live for another three years and then, 'I drop on the floor like my brother. Just fall on the floor and die'.

In general death itself was not feared by the women in this study, whatever their ethnic background or faith. The women told us:

I am not frightened. (Polish woman, aged 72)

148

I have to die soon. This July I am 80. Oh boy! I think the best time is now for me. (Polish woman)

I am not scared. (African-Caribbean woman, aged 69)

I don't think I am frightened about dying ... I feel so long as I can carry on as I am and doing what I am doing, it will happen and that will be it. But I don't think I am frightened of dying. (white middle-class, 66-year-old, Catholic participant)

Similar sentiments were uttered time and time again. However, although death itself might not be feared, the path to it was a real cause for concern. Many women echoed the view of one of our participants who declared, 'I want to die in good health'. An Indian contributor said that she wanted to 'go' before she was 'too old and frail to move around'. There was a general fear, as has been seen elsewhere in this study, of becoming a burden and an encumbrance on kin. This was particularly strong among our participants from the Indian sub-continent. As one of them put it:

We don't want to stay in bed and rot like, you know. I am praying every day for this. [I] want to die peacefully not ... life in bed and then no one wants to know, you know ... have to wait for death like. You don't want to carry on like.

Another said:

I am praying every day for this. I want to die peacefully not a life in bed and then no one wants to know you.

Two of our Hindu participants, aged 58 and 60, who were living with their husbands and who had come to the UK via Uganda, expressed similar views:

If I live, I pray with God. I work myself. I do my job myself. I can bath myself. I praying like this. If God wants, I pray I don't want to live.

We'd rather die with dignity.

Many other women also spoke about dying 'peacefully' and 'with dignity', and these were clearly very important aspects of their acceptance of death. Most of the Polish women who were Catholics though, while also concerned about having a dignified death, felt that they should live their lives to the end, even if they could do absolutely nothing – not even raise an eyelid, so to speak. Many also expressed strong fears about and antipathy towards euthanasia. As one said:

> We believe in God and we don't want any injections for death. We wait until we die naturally ... We don't worry. If we are very poorly and we want to die, we pray that we die and we die. If it is in Holland let that be. But not in England. Not in Polish community.

Speaking of what she regarded as dignity in death, a 77-year-old expressed concern that if you were regarded as a burden or in pain, doctors might try to assist or hasten the dying process:

> Dying with dignity ... lessening pain and dying with dignity. Not to be killed ... [a]lthough, of course, everyone has to die. But I would like to be a person through the death, more human like. Not to be killed like a dog.

Yet another repeated:

> Euthanasia. We are against abortion and against Euthanasia.

These views are clearly grounded in an unwavering faith. However, they may also reflect the extraordinary lives our Polish woman had led and survived as young people, together with the terrible things that they had seen. Some hoped to live a little longer to see their families grow and prosper. Others echoed the views of a participant with a heart problem, who told us that the later years had been 'the happiest time' of her life, now that she was living with her son and daughter in law. She hoped for 'a few more years'.

Many of our respondents viewed their later years in terms of preparation, or making ready, for the departure that would eventually follow. For example, a Polish widow, who had been a businesswoman, went on frequent pilgrimages. This seemed to her as a good way to travel as a woman alone, since she was able to meet some spiritual needs and prepare for the next life. Another, also a widow, had given her son sufficient money to pay for her funeral. A 64-year-old widowed Muslim was hoping to prepare for becoming older and subsequent death by undertaking Hajj, the Islamic pilgrimage to Mecca, 'with God's help'. A black Caribbean participant, who is a member of the Church of Jesus Christ of the Latter Day Saints, indicated:

That's how I see the future. Yes. Preparing myself, yeah, that when that time come, I can meet my Saviour, you know what I mean [laughs]. So I'm happy now. I'm really happy.

Some of the Indian participants were engaging in good works because this would, for them as Hindus, determine their next life. As one explained;

I believe this life is not everything. We've got other life also ... If we do good things in this life, then we get better life in future. Next life.

Further,

Future life is if you are still living. But next life is after death. Good place involves heaven. If you have done bad things then you get hell, just like you say.

Going on to explain transmigration in the Hindu faith, in which one might be reborn as any creature, she described how:

Hindus believe in life after death ... [It] might not be the same body we got. Might be cat, might be dog. Animals, worms, anything.

Another Hindu woman was preparing for her own transmigration. An interpreter told us how she:

goes to the temple every day in the morning but in summer time she goes at night. She prays at home as well and sings hymns [bhajans]. She wakes up at 6 am and prays, reads from her Gujarati book, which is a holy book and she sings hymns every morning. Religion is more important to her since getting older. After death, whatever she is doing now [in the way of good works and deeds will influence her future life], she will be reborn in a better environment.

This woman made a donation after an earthquake in Gujarat and she also gave some money to the community centre where older people including herself meet. This donation paid for lunch for everyone. She explained via the interpreter that whatever she is doing now will influence her next life and that she will be reborn in a better condition. Others also described how they 'tried' to do good things.

A minority though felt that there was no preparation that could be made. For instance, one Hindu participant had a more fatalistic attitude, saying:

Whatever is coming we have to face, you know. You can't prepare. I don't know how long I live, you know. No and what my position after five year, I don't know.

Many of the Muslim women in this study also were preparing for death by praying and reading holy books. Since some of these women were very isolated, these activities also provided comfort in 'this life'. Many of them lived something of a cloistered existence and, like some of the older Hindu women, they were unable to speak English. In a Muslim community, where kin is all important (Afshar 1989a), this isolation was almost a form of bereavement. For example, one very devout 80-year-old Muslim from Pakistan, who had only arrived in the UK when she was aged 62 and could not speak English, explained through an interpreter how she wanted her next life to be 'good' and how she only thinks about her next life now and hopes that it is not anything worse than what she has currently.

Some of the white women also had notions of living on after death, mainly through having brought up children and being associated with their activities, and then through their children's children and so on. Such tendencies have been noted by others (Walter 1999). The middle-class women especially, who were busy living full lives, were engaged in lots of social activities and had a lot of independence, talked about death in more distant ways than those from the minority ethnic groups. Some saw death as a practical problem for those who survived. One of our respondents talked about the death of a local woman, whose children had to sell the family house to pay death duties. This meant that the family could no longer get together on a regular basis and had to rent a suitable place to be able to meet once a year. There were worries about property and inheritance in this regard. Another, a retired teacher aged 72 and still living with her husband, spoke of how, obviously, one of them would die first and of how they had arranged how the survivor would be able to support themselves in terms of nursing, nursing homes 'and that sort of thing'. Another worried about potential isolation, if her husband was to die first, as he was the one who drove the car. Yet another explained how she viewed death with optimism, as she expected to meet all her friends again in the next life and what an enjoyable experience this would be. This constitutes an example of a form of personalized religion or spirituality, discussed in the previous chapter. Although she described herself as not 'being religious', she too believes in a form of afterlife. As she explained:

> Well, I wouldn't say it was a religious belief, it's just something I find helpful, in that I didn't believe in going ... well, I do believe in going to heaven, or whatever it is, to see people you have met beforehand because I didn't see the point in living, if you didn't go back and meet people again that you have met over your whole life.

The women in this study appeared to approach their own, possibly impending, death with equanimity. They expressed little fear and instead, depending on their faith and cultural allegiance, had striven to prepare for what was regarded as an inevitable eventuality and outcome. Buoyed by the religious and other principles to which they adhered, these women exhibit strength, stoicism and tenacity. They are in various ways both spiritually and practically preparing themselves for the end of their lives, at least in this incarnation of it. They do so, not only with fortitude, but for many, due to spiritual support, with happiness and optimism, as well as with resolution.

Widowhood

Over half of the participants in this study were widowed. In fact, generally, widowhood is the norm for older women worldwide, as well as in the UK. Using figures collected for the 2001 Census, the ONS (2004) suggests that nearly half of all women aged 65 and over in the UK are widows, rising to four-fifths at the age of 85 and over. In contrast, over three-quarters of men aged 65–9 are married. This falls to 60 percent by their early 80s, but even in their late 80s, half of the men in this age group remain married (ONS 2004). The reasons for this gender difference lie in the fact that women tend to partner men who are older than themselves. Because men on average die earlier than women, this means that losing a partner tends to be a feminized experience.

Losing a spouse is the most significant kind of bereavement to occur in later life. However, there is a paucity of material exploring this experience and virtually none of it is in relation to minority ethnic groups (Chambers 2000; Arber et al. 2003; Chambers 2005). Bennett, who has done most to put widowhood on the academic and policy agenda in the UK, found that it can profoundly affect both mental health and morale (1997a, b). It also influences social participation and relationships (Thuen 1997). Women are generally thought to cope better than men, due to a stronger female support network and what has been dubbed the 'society of widows', and research indicates that both genders believe that men fare worse than women (Bennett 2002). Bennett and Morgan (1992) have identified two distinct areas that affect later life widowhood. These are the bereavement *per se* and the transition to a single widowed status. Further, it has also been suggested that traditional stage theories of bereavement (e.g., Kubler-Ross's phases of: denial; anger; bargaining; depression; and, finally, acceptance/letting go) are less useful than had previously been thought (Kubler-Ross 1970; Bennett and Bennett 2001). Lopata (1996), for instance, raises the issue of whether approaching bereavement in such a way might hinder the adoption of the new widowhood role.

Loss of a spouse may lead to a real or perceived loss of status. It may mean having to learn to undertake new tasks about the house. It can involve losing contact with friends and bring about loneliness and depression (Bennett and Vidal-Hall 2000; Bennett and Bennett 2001). Keeping busy has been found to be an important aspect of widowed life, providing structure to the day, some meaning to life and an active means of coping. Somewhat obviously, a relationship has been found between length of time since being bereaved, coping and emotional adjustment (Bennett et al. 2005).

Becoming a widow had been a terrible shock to most of the women in this study, while a few had dealt with the experience with a degree of equanimity. For the majority it had meant the loss of the most important remnants of a lifetime, of past times, ideas and shared perspectives. Most of our participants experienced widowhood as a traumatic demarcation between a time that was 'then' and a time that was 'now'. Some had lost their husbands at very young ages and had had to struggle hard to bring up young children. A typical example was a Muslim woman from Pakistan, who had been widowed aged 16 with a 10-month-old baby, and had subsequently had to live with her parents. She said that being a widow has depressed her so much throughout her life that she tends to stay inside her house and prays in order to cope with it. She said that she:

started to feel old after my husband's died; from 16 until now for me life is old age.

Another Muslim woman originally from Bangladesh said that, following the death of her husband, she felt 'very very old and had no enthusiasm for nothing'.

Widowhood at a young age for women from the Asian subcontinent often resulted in the loss of independence. It proved more difficult to establish themselves as an independent source of authority within the kin group. They had become dependent on male relatives at an early age. Where the kinship networks themselves had begun to fracture, they felt themselves to be cast into isolation, with relatively little support or care. Some of our participants from the Indian subcontinent remembered that their mothers had considered Sati or widow-burning to be a norm. Although this no longer applied to them, they continued to accept to some extent the ascribed values of widowhood as both a blight and a burden.

Alongside the traumatic emotional loss, widowhood had also deprived many of those who had experienced it at younger ages of access to resources. This was particularly true of those migrants who did not speak English and who had left their husbands in charge of the myriad of officialdom and bureaucracy that had to be dealt with in the host country. A Muslim respondent told us through an interpreter that she continued over two decades to miss her husband and his companionship. She felt that she had lost control:

> the last 20 years for her, since her husband passed, have been no good. She has money problems. She feels she is locked inside the house. If she wants to go somewhere she has to get a taxi but she can't afford to do this.

Some of the less-well-off inner-city white women had also faced the harsh material effects of widowhood. One told us:

> I brought five kids up on this estate when my husband died. I had five children and I went through it.

The actual moment of the death of a husband had been lodged indelibly in the memory of some widows. For instance, a black Caribbean woman, who had been married for 40 years, remembered how:

Just before he died, you know, five minutes before he died, he was waiting for me. I went to the bathroom and I came back and I held him there, you know. He just died in my arms … I couldn't cry because I felt like crying because that means I'm giving up, so when he died and he died in my arms and he says to me 'I love you' and I said to him 'do you know who I am?' and he said 'Yeah'. He said 'you're my J'. He didn't talk because the cancer were [affecting] his throat. He said 'you're my J' and I say to him 'you love me?' and he said yeah'. So he give me a kiss then. He put his face up and give me a kiss and he put his hand up and he held me and he said to me, 'don't worry sweetheart, everything will be alright. Don't worry. Don't worry.' And then I just said, 'God bless his soul' and he just fall out and die in my arms.

Subsequently, J found it extremely difficult to cope. She was ill and unable to eat:

Yes and a few weeks when you get really, really poorly and I had to go to the doctor … I couldn't sleep, you know. I couldn't sleep … I said I didn't want any sedative or anything like that. I said I want to be in control. And he said to me, 'You haven't mourned your husband's death and you haven't cried enough and unless you can do that'. Anyway he gave me some minor little tablets to relax me a little bit.

Similarly, an Indian participant described how:

I became very, very ill, very, very disturbed, stressed, out very depressed. I went into a coma for twenty-six hours.

A Polish woman reported how, after the death of her second husband, she had decided to take her own life:

I been so bad depressed I wanted to die because my husband die, my second husband die. First my husband die. He was 54 when my son was only 16. Then, after a few years, I marry again and another die with heart. Heart attack just drop. And I live a few years by my own and something happen, I just want to die. And I take overdose tablets. Sat down on the floor in the kitchen and I collect few weeks. I collect tablets, you know, and my son been married already then and every evening he telephone to me 'Are you alright? Are you alright?' or something. He would telephone every night. So when he telephone and I not answer, he called to my house and found me on the floor unconscious. And I was in hospital … for some days and after straight away they took me to …

Another woman, who had lost her husband three years previously, still could not talk about him without feeling very upset:

Sometimes I feel really awful. That it would be better if I die ... I think. I don't bother about my health now. No. I am now I don't bother. Of course, I have children and grandchildren but I, sometimes, I wonder why I am living [gives a little embarrassed laugh].

One of the Pakistani women wailed with grief, some 20 or more years after the death of her husband, when talking about it at one of our focus groups. It was clearly the worst thing that had happened to her.

The pain and sorrow of widowhood did not recognize boundaries of creed, ethnicity or colour. All found it equally difficult to cope with the death of their husbands. One of the white rural participants explained in relation to her religious beliefs how:

I can't get anything out of it. I can't tell you why. When my husband died, I expected to get a lot out of it but, then, all I could think of was why did he have to go at 53 and I couldn't grasp anything to do with it.

A white working-class woman found it difficult to come to terms with her husband's death and could not part from his clothes.

And still getting rid of his clothes and all his belongings that was very hard for me. People used to say to me 'Get rid of it. Get rid of his things'. I said 'I can't'. I couldn't go in his drawer and touch nothing. I couldn't but I had to do it in the end. What the kids wanted, they took and I took it to Cancer Research. So my sons took some and take down for me. I did it in stages. And he took them to Cancer Research and Heart Foundation, you know. Somebody will get something out of it because you need more research.

After five months this contributor reported that she was just beginning to come to terms with her husband's death and had started tending his grave.

Even for those who had managed to contain feelings of grief mainly within themselves, the death of a husband remained extremely hard to cope with such was the sense of loss that had been carved. One black Caribbean woman commented that the quality of her life would have improved dramatically had her husband still been alive. Another explained:

And, you know, I can see him time and time again, you know. The same thing. Where he sat by the window and looking out.

Other women also reported how they can still visualize their partners sitting in a favourite chair, standing in a particular place or engaged in a particular activity. One of the middle-class white women indicated that it was the little things that she found most difficult to cope with. For instance, she had found a calendar on which her husband had made entries. Seeing his handwriting, and remembering the events that he had noted, was distressing. Respondents also described how they found solace in talking to the husbands who had passed on. A Polish woman, whose husband had died eight years previously, wishes he was still here and misses his company:

> I talk to him. I believe that he hears me. He listens to me and I sort of pray and thank him for all the good years we had together … I really believe almost that he looks after me. I dream now and again about him and I believe in my dreams.

An African-Caribbean widow spoke of how she told her husband when she was going to bed and said 'good morning' to him when she woke up. She gets comfort from talking to him.

Other participants got solace from having their husband's photographs around the house. Although this could sometimes bring back painful memories, the presence of these pictures also served in recalling happy occasions and in fuelling memories and keeping them alive. This was at once both a source of sorrow and a comfort.

Others felt that widowhood deprived them of the rhythm of their lives, of their closest friendship and, for some, of a reason to live. As the participant whose husband died of throat cancer explained, parting was difficult and she started the role of widow in a state of denial:

> We were married forty years … And we know each other a long, long time before that. Like we more or less been together all our lives. And it's very hard for me to readjust, you know, because I have to accept that he's not coming back. That is the only way I can carry on. You know, it's like its not happening. I know he's dead but, you know, it's like this is not happening, you know.

A white woman felt her greatest achievement during the first year after her husband's death was survival, since she felt so very low and in despair:

> The first year was the hardest. All those occasions, like Christmas and birthdays and Sunday dinners, when he was not there.

An African-Caribbean contributor explained:

I miss him terribly. My life is not the same but I have to readjust. You see, I have to go on living but the quality of life is not one that I wanted because I'm having to make do. Now I'm a bit older and I got more sense and more settled and you can think about what you're doing you know. But you don't have to think about anyone else. If your children were little, I would be thinking of them. I'm the last person I would be thinking about.

Some widows had found help in their faith. One widow, who is a Muslim, found some solace in religious rituals and gatherings:

We had a, a lovely gathering yesterday in my house. I had about 30 women in the house. They came and prayed for my husband ... . I cooked, my daughters and my daughters-in-law cooked a lot of food and it was very nice food and everybody shared. We had a lovely time. It was very. We really had a lovely time and it was good while everybody's there, when everybody goes ... .

An African-Caribbean woman, who had found the loss of her husband almost impossible to bear, was nevertheless pleasantly surprised by the support of friends and neighbours:

I can tell you when my husband die I never see those people do things like that for me. Round the area they got money. White people, yeah. Oh, they brought the money anyway. They raise that money. So I said I didn't want no flowers for him. So I raise that money to send to Intensive Care, you know. Yes. So I raise £200 and I send it to intensive care. You see, that's where he was. And I say ... when the people bring the money for me I start to cry. I never know they would do that. All the people. Yes, and the children even they Pakistan or Indian, they still nice. They still come and telling me, asking me if I want anything. I can't say nothing but 'God Bless.'

A similarity across all groups was the loss of identity felt when a partner died. Some said that they felt that they no longer knew who they were and talked of having to rebuild their identity. In addition to the loss of a friend and a partner, widowhood could make women into 'displaced homemakers'. Those who had concentrated on their domestic duties and left the management of their affairs to their husbands experienced a double sense of loss. One said:

And like I said ... my life is completely change you know, completely. Completely ... It is a big issue. You know, you plan your life when you retire. You know what we are going to do. We're going to go and set ourselves up for retirement and the next thing you know you single which is devastating. Your quality of life for me is gone.

Many of our participants had been comforted by their family and had found the strength to continue but were also proud of having managed without much assistance. An 80-year-old, inner-city-living, white respondent told us:

Well I never had any sort of counselling when I lost my husband. It was straight back to work and I got £1.50 a week pension, and if, when there was a shortage of work and we used to have to go and sign on, that £1.50 a week was taken off me. And it was classed as income for income tax. That was £1.50 a week, so I had to work to keep meself.

Coping sometimes meant continuing with existing plans and trying to fulfil the wishes of the deceased. Another inner-city woman's husband had died six weeks before their daughter's marriage. She felt that she would let him down if she did not continue with the wedding. Despite her grief she decided to go on and convinced her daughter that it was the best solution:

It was a bit awkward but he would have wanted her to continue. She didn't want to at the time but he'd have wanted her to so, you can't do that. It's hard. It is hard.

Some of our participants had rekindled old interests and/or had found new ones. Others preferred to maintain the life that they had shared with their partners. Some felt that they could not live surrounded by happy memories of their life with their husbands and others felt that they could not move away from them. A number decided to remain in the homes that they had shared with their partners; others chose to move on. Such decisions depended on individual responses to loss and are not, on the basis of this research, easily generalizable.

It is clear that while women eventually coped with widowhood, the majority required some personal and practical support. Many said that that it was only the friendship of one or two people that had helped them survive immediately after the death. Although close friends and family members are important at this time, the women also needed someone outside of this network to talk to. A number indicated that they found it difficult to talk of their grief with close friends and family because they had also known their husbands and they did not want to upset them. For instance, an African-Caribbean woman, who had been recently widowed, talked of how she was grieving but felt that she could not talk to her friends about it. She had to remain cheerful, looking 'like the next sunny day but crying inside'. She said:

> I just say 'Oh I'm okay' ... because they get depressed as well. I just carry on. The nights are worse ... And every sound you thinking .... .

Similarly, another told us:

> I will say to them [her children] 'don't worry about me', even though I feel very depressed and that. I don't tell them any more.

A white inner-city woman explained that:

> Um, after I lost him, I was fine outside and I had my dull face in the house by myself. I wouldn't give in. I wouldn't take it out with me ... I did a lot of grieving in the house on my own not ... even with my family, my two sons and my daughter. They knew I was but I wouldn't let it go. I needed ... when I was on my own.

Some felt that they had to cope with the grief on their own in order to keep the family together. Another 60-year-old African-Caribbean woman, who had been recently widowed, felt that she had to cope alone:

> I have to do this on my own, you see. They all have their own life and I don't want to be dependent on them, because if you have a family and you're not spending enough time with your family that can cause a lot of [trouble], because they will be the falling out and 'you're paying too much attention to your mum' and my husband he stated in the will that he [the son] should look after me. I try to tell them I can look after myself. If there's anything I need and I can get the money together, I pay somebody to do it.

Support offered by friends, relatives and faith communities to widows was one of the important ways of dealing with their loss and solitude. One of our participants felt that a bereavement counsellor, who would be prepared to visit women in their homes, would improve this situation. Another had moved away from the Anglican Church to the Church of Jesus Christ and Latter Day Saints (popularly called Mormon):

> 'cause they're always there for you. Somebody always comes to see you, specially if you're on your own.

The widows in this study reported that the time of day that was most difficult for them was in the evening. This was when, if living alone, as most of them did, doors were shut, curtains drawn and feelings of isolation and loneliness began to set in. This was particularly the case during the dark nights of the winter. A focus group of women from the Commonwealth of Dominica explained how it was 'terrible when it gets dark early in the evenings' and 'the worst time is winter. Dark night and everything. Its terrible'. They also reported how, 'it looks like a very, very long day', which was a problem because, 'Yeah, night all the time isn't it. You can't go out and see people'.

The Polish widows reported that, 'in the evenings it is lonely. The evenings are very lonely, you know' and how it was 'a bit sad when you are on your own. Those long dark evenings'. Further:

> You can't go out because you don't dare. You don't dare go out in the evening. So, as soon as its getting dark, we just close our windows and doors and stay at home because you don't dare going out.

A white working-class widow, whose friends had been encouraging her to go out with them, said that one of the most difficult things was returning home on her own. As she put it, 'what I hated most of all was coming back in the house ... that was the terrible part'.

The Bangladeshi, Indian and Pakistani widows were extremely distressed and burdened by their current status and most of them had retreated into their faith and prayer. Some of the women from the other groups, however, although still grieving, did express that they had also experienced a degree of liberation in their newly found position. One 73-year-old Jamaican-born contributor said that she was enjoying both retirement and widowhood:

> When you live with a husband, you never have enough control [laughs loudly] because when your husband ... well let's say partner ... you got to think of them, so you can't say I'm going to do this or that, so you're not in full control, I think. So long as you're not single you're not in full

control. What is good about my life? I've retired. I've worked. I've done my bit for England. And I've retired. I have lots of aches and pains, as you know it comes with age. But I feel very happy, fulfilled.

Other African-Caribbean women were playing greater roles in their centres, communities and church than they had done previously, as were those in the Polish group. The white women, especially the more affluent rural ones, were using their extra time to undertake various kinds of voluntary work. In this respect, they were developing new skills and taking on new roles to the extent that they sometimes surprised themselves in terms of finding out about their abilities. For example, one described how she had been asked to become president of the local WI:

I said 'oh no, it's not the job I can do, I would rather be washing up in the kitchen'. You know, it's not my kind of job ... and so I was kind of talked into it ... and, actually, now I have got into it, I quite enjoy it, just at the local level, you know.

Another told how, when her husband was dying, he said that he was worried that she would not be able to continue running their guest house without him. However, she persevered and:

I think I have achieved that, without thinking that I would. If anyone had said to me, 'right you will be running a guest house one day', I think I would have been quite frightened.

Thus, even in the adversity of widowhood, it is possible to find the strength and determination to take on new responsibilities and widen existing horizons.

Conclusion

Death, dying and the experience of bereavement had been significant for the women in this study throughout their life course. Events that had taken place during the Second World War had been particularly important, with references to them peppering their accounts of their lives and how they see themselves today. Bereavement is painful and distressing at any time and our participants spoke movingly about the loss of a range of family and kin members, as well as friends. They were prepared to speak openly about these experiences of loss, as well as about how they viewed, and what they would wish for, regarding their own demise. However, it was concerning the death of husbands that the widowed women spoke most. Nothing had prepared them, even when they had known in advance that partners were dying, for the trauma and pain of that experience which, for many, lasted years and years after the event and which, of course, never entirely ceases. Some of their accounts of their feelings, illustrations of which have been offered in this chapter, were extremely harrowing.

However, in the conclusion to this chapter, we now need to make an admission. For, initially, we had not intended to research widowhood and had not included consideration of it in our research proposal and preparations. Like other researchers of later life, death had not been regarded as a central concern. It was the widows themselves in this study who made sure that we understood how shocking and emotionally distressing the death of a husband was and, further, how these emotions, although usually abating, never disappear entirely and could suddenly reappear years later, with renewed force. Such strong waves of emotional feeling were not just due to losing a loved one, partner and friend but were exacerbated for many by the change of status that ensued, leaving women to look for new roles and activities in lives that had been changed. This was particularly the case for our participants who originated from the Indian subcontinent. Although respected as older women, they felt that their standing was somewhat diminished by their widowhood to an extent that most had retreated into their religions.

It is, therefore, important that those who study later life acknowledge the significance of being a widow and the changes that this brings (Chambers 2000; Arber et al. 2003; Chambers 2005). Looking at widowhood from the psychological perspective of stages of grief, coping and adjustment strategies and counselling the individual are important in providing support to those dealing with loss. However, widowhood is also a rite of passage, often indicating that one has advanced quite a long way along the road, which is life. The social implications of this, particularly in terms of service provision and policy implementation, require much greater acknowledgement and understanding.

9

Conclusions

Conclusions to books can involve different kinds of endings. Sometimes authors provide an overview of the book's content or they may offer a summary of the main findings or a guide to the central arguments. However, since we have provided brief conclusions to each chapter, it does not seem necessary to engage in such repetition here. Rather, we intend to do two things. The first is to suggest four general ways in which we hope that this book has contributed to a better understanding of age, gender and ethnicity. The second is to look more specifically at some issues in relation to the life course perspective where we hope that this book might also have made a contribution.

In this book we have sought to contribute to understanding the relationships between gender, ethnicity and aging in the lives of older women. We were interested, in particular, in how different cultures and contexts resonate through the meanings and experiences of later life and the implications of these for the women themselves. In this we hope to have made a contribution in a number of areas. The first of these is in terms of later life research *per se*, where the substantive considerations arising from our fieldwork extend empirical knowledge about later life, in general, and in relation to women and ethnicity in particular. This signals the importance of looking at difference and diversity as part of the process of reaching a better understanding of the lives of older people. Older lives are not simply about *either* gender *or* ethnicity but can involve complex interrelations between the two. However, this is not just the case for minority ethnic women as studies usually assume. For many of the older white women who participated in this study, their identity was, in part, based on their ethnicity as white and their nationality as English. The significance of whiteness as an ethnicity for older people has yet to be explored very far in the literature.

A second area that we have attempted to address in the book is in connection with some of the theoretical and conceptual issues that were discussed both in Chapter 3 and indeed throughout the book itself. These are concerned with the most appropriate ways in which to frame questions, position and make sense of research, without unconsciously using concepts, ideas and assumptions that are derived from work with white British subjects. In the same way that anthropologists and those working in the area of development studies ask questions as to how far across the world concepts and approaches can legitimately be transported, these questions also need to be asked in the West. Specifically, to what extent is it acceptable to use concepts and perspectives, drawn from one particular cultural setting, in others that may have different norms and values? What needs to be done to interrogate our often unconsciously held, cultural assumptions and produce more nuanced understanding? How can we ensure that the approaches we use are ethnically sensitive?

Third, in discussing the lives and experiences of older women, we hope to signal to those involved in women's/gender/feminist studies the need for these women to be put firmly on their agenda. This is not simply to reduce the invisibility of women who are older, although a case can certainly be made for this. It is also because, as we hope this book has demonstrated, their rich stories make an important contribution to our knowledge of gender and gender relations in this early part of the 21st century.

Fourth, and for reasons similar to those just discussed, those who are involved in studying 'race' and ethnicity would also benefit from being able to include discussions about older minority ethnic people's position and views. This would offer a more rounded picture of ethnic differences and inequalities in the UK today. In other words, there are synergies to be made here in terms of cross-cutting effort and cross-cutting research and in breaching what are often constituted as separate fields of study and research ghettos. It is interesting to note that Blakemore and Boneham (1994) expressed similar sentiments in *Age, Race and Ethnicity*, while also warning that dominant ways of thinking in social gerontology would need to be problematized when taking account of ethnic difference. Yet we hazard to suggest that not much has changed in the intervening years since the latter book's publication.

In addition to these more general aspects, other more particular issues have emerged during the course of the book. The first of these relates to the significance of the life course and of events and experiences in connection with this to the older women in our study. In one sense there is nothing novel about this, since many others have also written about the importance of adopting a life course perspective (as opposed to that of the life cycle) when studying later life. As Hareven, who is closely associated with the development of the concept, put it:

> Rather than focusing on stages of the life cycle, the life course approach is concerned with how individuals and families made their transitions into those different stages. Rather than viewing any one stage of life, such as childhood, youth, and old age, or any group in isolation, it is concerned with an understanding of the place of that stage in an entire life continuum. (1982: xiii)

The emphasis here is on flexibility, variation and transition. Not only is this visible in the lives of our participants, but the extent to which the processes that they have previously been through have helped to mould who they are today is also very clear. Their identities are influenced not just by current roles and experiences but by the particular journeys that they have taken through life. We are trying to emphasize here that being an older woman (or older person more generally for that matter) cannot just be read off from the here and now but is a reflexive process in which previous experiences and senses of identity are reassembled in the present to reinscribe the self. This means that identity in later life is not simply to be understood in relation to age *per se*, but is crucially linked to the past as well as to the future. The latter may be seen in our respondents' hopes for relationships with family and kin and aspirations for a good death. As we have seen, these are laced with concerns about independence and dignity and about not wanting to become either a nuisance or a burden.

It is clear, for example, that for the minority ethnic group women, the experience of migration has been crucial, since they were at pains to discuss this to a very great extent. This was not just because of the experiences of hardship, deprivation and racism, but the very process of migration itself was often traumatic involving, as it did, moving from one set of cultural norms, customs and ways of life to another that were different. As was discussed in Chapter 4, this was done with

no attempt made by the 'host' culture to provide guidance or information about what was to be expected or what sort of changes there
might be. Further, this migration process cannot simply be seen as a
one-off event and the status of migrant, although clearly diminishing,
does not completely disappear over time. This is because 'white' society
continues to ascribe the nomenclature 'migrant' to the women and
their construction as part of an ethnic minority also marginalizes them
and categorizes them as different. As we have shown, this came as a
huge shock to many. For the Polish women, their terrible wartime
experiences are also part of the life course that inscribes their current
selves. The war also features in some of the white women's accounts of
their life journey.

The life course trajectory also influences our older women's current
experiences and sense of self in other ways. For instance, it impinges on
past and present relationships with family and kin. It helps to shape
their experiences of health and well-being in later life. It informs their
ongoing involvement with religion, faith and spirituality. Our discussion of the latter in particular has underlined the extent to which most
of the older women in our study were guided by such beliefs. This was
the case even for those who we have described as 'believing and partially belonging'.

The research that has been discussed in this book illustrates the
complexities in analysing women's lives across different ethnicities and
religions. There are things that all our women share, some because of
their age and some due to their gender. There are dimensions that are
held in common due to ethnic background and faith and which,
thereby, differentiate them from those in other groups. Personal, as
well as group, biographies also affect women individually. Thus, later
life for women can be analysed in terms of its collective gendered
nature. It can be discussed in terms of group properties, for instance
ethnicity and religion, but one might also add socio-economic differences and other forms of diversity here. It may also be explored in
biographical terms, where collective and group elements will be steeped
with more particular individual histories and narratives.

We have also sought in this book to emphasize the dynamic and
intermingled relationship between notions of structure and agency.
For, while particular social and material factors obviously constitute
frameworks within which older women act, this does not mean that

their lives can be simply reduced to or read off from these. Rather, the participants upon whom we have focused are clearly active agents in their own lives. This is the case, even when it might not appear so to the casual observer, as with for example, some of the Asian women who had chosen to retreat into prayer.

In Chapter 3, we discussed our attempts to develop a post-gerontology, one which would explore how different cultures and systems of belief might contribute to well-being for older women and the pages that followed are the first steps of development in this direction. Further, we considered the utility of notions of empowerment and disempowerment. Here Rowlands' model of power-sharing was discussed (1998). The women in our study clearly had all elements of 'power over', 'power to', 'power with' and 'power from within' in their lives, although there were differences in terms of balance between these elements in relation to the extent, strength and degree of each. Some women were able to exercise quite a lot of 'power over' as evidenced for instance, by the more affluent white women who were involved in organizing and running local activities. Some women had significant amounts of 'power to', for example through their roles in the moral economy of kin. Other women were empowered through 'power with' as they were participating in collective activities with families, friends, and local and faith communities. Others had 'power from within' in terms of spirituality and prayer. The point is, however, that the types of power described here are not zero-sum and they are likely to expand exponentially or diminish depending on circumstances.

In relation to this, we also pointed out in Chapter 3 that there are different kinds of empowerment, that empowerment and disempowerment are relational, constituting a process rather than a given state, and that it is possible to be empowered and disempowered simultaneously and to different degrees in different aspects of one's life. So, for example, women who were widowed gained strength from friends and family and sometimes from religion. Those who got immense satisfaction from looking after grandchildren might also be restricted in others ways by lack of income. Others whose mobility was limited gained solace from more home-based activities such as cooking and sewing for family and friends, as well as from memories of past times. The point is that these women are not victims, although some of them do display degrees of vulnerability, nor are they coping with old age. They are instead living through aging and, as with every age group, the journey through which they are moving involves taking on certain kinds of life course baggage at particular moments in time.

Bibliography

Adam, B. (2004) *Time*. Cambridge: Polity.

Afshar, H. (1987) The Muslim concept of law, *International Encyclopedia of Comparative Law*. Tubingen: The Hague and Paris: J.C.B. Mohr.

Afshar H. (1989a) Gender roles and the 'moral economy of kin' among Pakistani women in West Yorkshire. *New Community* 15(2): 21125.

Afshar, H. (1989b) Education, hopes, expectations and achievements of Muslim women in West Yorkshire, *Gender and Education*, 1(3): 261–82.

Afshar, H. (1994) Values real and imaginary and their ascription to women: some remarks about growing up with conflicting views of self and society among Muslim families in West Yorkshire, in H. Afshar and M. Maynard (eds), *The Dynamics of Race and Gender*. London: Taylor & Francis.

Afshar, H., Aitken, R. and Franks, M. (2005a) Feminisms, Islamophobia and identities. Paper presented at the seminar on Social Justice and Multiculturalism: Tensions and Possibilities, York Council for Voluntary Service, 24 November.

Afshar, H., Aitken, R. and Franks, M. (2005b) Feminisms, Islamophobia and Identities, *Political Studies*, 53: 262–83.

Afshar H. Aitken R. and Franks M. (2006) 'Islamaphobia and women of Pakistani descent in Bradford: the crisis of ascribed and adopted identities, in Moghissi, H. (ed.) *Muslim Diaspora: Gender culture and identity*. London and New York: Routledge, pp.167–185.

Afshar, H. and Alikhan, F. (2002) Age and empowerment among slum dwelling women in Hyderabad, *Journal of International Development*, 14(8): 1153–61.

Afshar, H., Franks, M.; Maynard, M. and Wray, S. (2001) Empowerment, disempowerment and quality of life for older women, *Generations Review*, 11(4):12–13.

Afshar, H. Franks, M. Maynard, M. and Wray, S. (2002) Age and ethnicities: demystifying the myths, *ESRC Growing Older Programme Report*.

Age Concern (2000) *Black and Minority Ethnic Elders' Issues*. London: Age Concern.

Age Concern (2002) *Black and Minority Ethnic Elders' Issues*. London: Age Concern.

Age Concern (2007) *Older People in the United Kingdom*. London: Age Concern.

Ainlay, S. Singelton, C.J. Jr. and Swigert, V. (1992) Aging and religious participation: reconsidering the effects of health, *Journal for the Scientific Study of Religion*, 31(2): 175–88.

Allatt, P., Keil, T., Bryman, A. and Bytheway, B. (eds) (1987) *Women and the Life Cycle: Transitions and Turning-points*. London: Macmillan.

Andrews, G.R. (2001) Promoting health and function in an aging population. *British Medical Journal*, 322: 728–29.

Andrews, M. (1999) The seductiveness of agelessness, *aging and Society*, 19: 302–18.

Anthias, F. (2002) Where do I belong? Narrating collective identity and translocational positionality, *Ethnicities*, 2(4): 491–515.

Arber, S. (1998) Health, aging and older women, in L. Doyal, L. Harrison and P. Charlwood (eds) *Women and the National Health Service: A Case for Change?* Buckingham: Open University Press.

Arber, S. and Attias-Donfut, C. (2000) *The Myth of Generational Conflict: The Family and State in aging Societies*, London: Routledge.

Arber, S. and Cooper, H. (1999) Gender difference in health in later life: the new paradox? *Social Sciences and Medicine*, 48(1): 61–7.

Arber, S. and Cooper, H. (2000) Gender and inequalities in women's health across the life course, in E. Annandale and K. Hunt (eds), *Gender Inequalities in Health* Buckingham: Open University Press.

Arber, S., Davidson, K. and Ginn, J. (2003) Changing approaches to gender and later life, in S. Arber, K. Davidson and J. Ginn (eds), *Gender and aging*. Maidenhead, Berkshire: Open University Press.

Arber, S. and Evandrou, M. (eds) (1993a) *aging, Independence and the*

Life Course. London: Jessica Kingsley in association with the British Society of Gerontology.

Arber, S. and Evandrou, M. (1993b) Mapping the territory: aging, independence and the life course, in S. Arber and M. Evandrou (eds), *aging, Independence and the Life* Course, London: Jessica Kingsley.

Arber, S. and Ginn, J. (1991) *Gender and Later Life*, London: Sage

Aries, P. (1983) *The Hour of Our Death*, London: Peregrine

Arksey, H. and Knight, P. (1999) *Interviewing for Social Scientists*, London: Sage.

Armstrong, D. (1987) Silence and truth in death and dying, *Social Science and Medicine*, 24(8).

Armstrong, M. Jocelyn (2000) Older women's organization of friendship support networks: an African American-white American comparison, *Journal of Women and Aging*, 12 (1): 93–107

Arthur, S., Snape, D. and Dench, G. (2003) *The Moral Economy of Grandparenting*, London: National Centre for Social Research

Ballard, N. (2000) Panth, Kismet, Dham te Qaum: four dimensions in Punjabi religion, in P. Singh and S. Thandi (eds), *Punjabi Identity in a Global Context*, Delhi: Oxford University Press.

Barnes, M., Blom, A., Cox, K., Lessof, C. and Walker, A. (2006) *The Social Exclusion of Older People: Evidence from the First Wave of the English Longitudinal Study of aging (ELSA)*, London: HMSO.

Barnard, H. and Pettigrew, N. (2003) *Delivering Benefits and Services for Black and Minority Ethnic Older People*, DWP Report No. 201, CDS Leeds.

Barnes, H. and Taylor, R. (2006) *Work, Savings and Retirement Among Ethnic Minorities: A Qualitative Study*, Leeds: DWP

Batson, C.D., Schoenrade, P. and Ventis, W.L. (1993) *Religion and the Individual: A Social-psychological Perspective*, 2nd edn., New York: Oxford University Press.

Becker, G.S. (1976) *The Economic Approach to Human Behaviour*, Chicago: University of Chicago Press.

Beckford, J.A. (1999) The pragmatics of defining religion: the politics of defining religion in secular society: from a taken for granted institution to a contested resource, *Studies in the History of Religions*, 84: 23–40.

Beckford, J. and Walliss, J. (eds) (2006) *Theorizing Religion: Classical and Contemporary Debates.* Aldershot: Ashgate.

Bengtson, V.L. and Schaie, K.W. (eds) (1999) *The Handbook of Theories of Aging.* New York: Springer.

Bennett, K.M. (1997a) Widowhood in elderly women: the medium and long-term effects on mental and physical health, *Mortality,* 2(2): 137–48.

Bennett, K.M. (1997b) A longitudinal study of wellbeing in widowed women, *International Journal of Geriatric Psychiatry,* 2(1): 61–6.

Bennett, K.M. (2002) Social engagement as a precursor of mortality amongst people in later life, *Age and aging,* 31: 165–8.

Bennett, K.M. and Bennett, G. (2001) 'And there's always this great hole inside that hurts': an empirical study of bereavement in later life, *Omega,* 42(3): 237–51.

Bennett, K.M., Hughes, G.M. and Smith, P.T. (2005) The effects of strategy and gender on coping with widowhood, *Omega,* 51(1): 33–52.

Bennett, K.M. and Morgan, K. (1992) Health, social functioning and marital status: stability and change among recently widowed women, *International Journal of Geriatric Psychiatry,* 7(11): 813–17.

Bennett, K.M. and Vidal-Hall, S. (2000) Narratives of death: a qualitative study of widowhood in women in later life, *aging and Society,* 20(4): 413–28.

Berger, P. L. (1967) *The Sacred Canopy.* New York. Anchor Books, Doubleday.

Bernard, M. (2000) *Promoting Health in Old Age.* Buckingham: Open University Press.

Bernard, M. and Harding Davies, V. (2000) Our aging selves: reflecting on growing older, in M. Bernard, J. Phillips, L. Machin and V. Harding Davies (eds), *Women aging: Changing Identities, Challenging Myths,* London: Routledge.

Bernard, M. and Meade, K. (eds) (1993a) *Women Come of Age.* London: Edward Arnold.

Bernard, M. and Meade, K. (1993b) A third age lifestyle for older women?, in M. Bernard and K. Meade (eds), *Women Come of Age.* London: Edward Arnold.

Berthoud, R. (2002) Poverty and prosperity among Britain's ethnic minorities, *Benefits,* 10(33): 3–8.

Biggs, S. (1993) *Understanding aging: Images, Attitudes and Professional*

Practice. Buckingham: Open University Press.

Biggs, S. (1997) Choosing not to be old: masks, bodies and identity management in later life, *aging and Society*, 17(5): 533–53.

Biggs, S., Lowenstein, A. and Hendricks, J. (eds) (2003) *The Need for Theory: Critical Approaches to Social Gerontology*. Amityville, NY: Baywood.

Birren, J.E. and Bengston, V.L. (1988) *International Perspectives on Families, Aging and Social Support*. New York: Springer.

Black, H.K. (1999) Life as gift: spiritual narratives of elderly African-America women living in poverty, *Journal of Aging Studies*, 13(4): 441–55.

Blakemore, K. and Boneham, M. (1994) *Age, Race and Ethnicity: A Comparative Approach*. Buckingham: Open University Press.

Blakemore, K. (1996) *Age Race and Ethnicity: A Comparative Approach*. Buckingham: Open University Press.

Bloch, A. (2002) *The Migration and Settlement of Refugees in Britain*. Houndsmills: Palgrave Macmillan.

Bowling, B. (1990) *Elderly People from Ethnic Minorities: A Report on Four Projects*, London: Age Concern Institute of Gerontology, Kings College.

Bracken, P.J. and Petty, C. (1998) *Rethinking the Trauma of War*. Oxford: Free Association Books.

Bracken, P. and Thomas, P. (2001) Post-psychiatry: a new direction for mental health, *British Medical Journal*, 322: 724–7.

Bradford Health Authority. Available at www.bradford-ha.nhs.uk (accessed 23 October 2001).

Bradley, H. (1996) *Fractured Identities*. Cambridge: Polity Press.

Brannen, J., Moss, P. and Mooney, A. (2005) *Working and Caring Over the Twentieth Century: Change and Continuity in Four-generation Families*. London: Palgrave Macmillan.

Brasher, B.E. (1998) *Godly Women: Fundamentalism and Female Power*, New Brunswick, NJ: Rutgers University Press.

Braybon, G. and Summerfield, P. (1986) *Out of the Cage: Women's Experiences of Two World Wars*. London: Pandora Press.

Brewer, M., Browne, J., Emmerson, C. et al. (2007) *Pensioner Poverty over the Next Decade: What Role for Tax and Benefit Reform?* London: Institute for Fiscal Studies.

Brown, C. (2001) *The Death of Christian Britain*. London: Routledge.

Brown, H. et al. (eds) (1999) *White? Women.* York: Raw Nerve Books Ltd.

Browne, C.V. (1998) *Women, Feminism and Aging.* New York: Springer.

Bulmer, M. and Solomos, J. (eds) (2004) *Researching Race and Racism.* London: Routledge.

Bunton, R. and Burrows, R. (1995). Consumption and health in the 'epidemiological' clinic of late modern medicine, in R. Bunton, S. Nettleton and R. Burrows (eds), *The Sociology of Health Promotion: Critical Analyses of Consumption, Lifestyle and Risk,* London: Routledge.

Burholt, V. (2004) The settlement patterns and residential histories of older Gujaratis, Punjabis and Sylhetis in Birmingham, England, *Aging and Society,* 24: 383–409.

Butt, J. and Moriarty, J. (2004) Social support and ethnicity in old age, in A. Walker and C. Hagan Hennessy (eds), *Growing Older: Quality of Life in Old Age.* Maidenhead: Open University Press.

Butt, J. and Moriarty, J. (2005) Quality of life and support among older people from different ethnic groups, in A. Walker with S. Northmore (eds), *Growing Older in a Black and Ethnic Minority Group,* London: Age Concern.

Bytheway, B. (1995) *Ageism.* Buckingham: Open University Press.

Calasanti, T.M. and Slevin, K.F. (2001) *Gender, Social Inequalities and Aging,* Walnut Creek, CA: AltaMira Press.

Carr, D. (2003) A 'good death' for whom? Quality of spouse's death and psychological distress among older widowed persons, *Journal of Health and Social Behaviour,* 44(2): 215–32.

Chambers, P. (2000) Widowhood in later life, in M. Bernard, J. Phillips, L. Machin and V. Harding Davies (eds), *Women and aging,* London: Routledge.

Chambers, P. (2005) *Older Widows and the Lifecourse: Multiple Narratives of Hidden Lives.* Aldershot: Ashgate.

Chivallon, C.D. (2001) Society and space, *Environment and Planning,* 19: 461–83.

Chohan, S. (2001) The lure of the Baba, unpublished paper presented at the BASR/EASR annual conference, Faculty of Divinity, Cambridge University, 10–13 September.

Cole, T.R. (1992) *The Journey of Life: A Cultural History of Aging in America.* New York: Springer.

Coleman, P. (1994) Adjustment in later life, in J. Bond, P. Coleman and S. Peace (eds), *aging in Society*. London: Sage.

Coleman, P.G., McKiernan, F., Mills, M.A. and Speck, P. (2002) Spiritual belief and quality of life: the experience of older bereaved spouses, *Quality of aging*, 3: 20–6.

Collier, J.F. and Yanagisako, S.J. (eds) (1990) *Gender and Kinship*, Stanford: Stanford University Press.

Cooper, H. and Arber, S. (2003) Ethnicity and inequalities in older women's health, in F. Poland and G. Boswell (eds), *Women's Minds/Women's Bodies: Interdisciplinary Perspectives*. London: Macmillan.

Cook, J., Maltby, T. and Warren, L. (2004) A participatory approach to older women's quality of life, in A. Walker and C. Hagan Hennessey (eds), *Growing Older: Quality of Life in Old Age*. Maidenhead: Open University Press.

Cornwall, M. (1989) Faith development of men and women over the lifespan, in S. Bahl and E. Peterson (eds), *aging and the Family*. Lexington, MA: Lexington Books/D.C. Heath.

Craig, G., Dornan, P. with Bradshaw, J., Garbutt, R., Mumtaz, S., Syed, A. and Ward, A. (2003) *Underwriting Citizenship for Older People*. Hull: University of Hull.

Cumming, E. and Henry, W.E. (1966) *Growing Old: The Process of Disengagement*. New York: Basic Books.

Davidson, K., Warren, L. and Maynard, M. (2005) Social involvement: aspects of gender and ethnicity, in A. Walker (ed.) *Understanding Quality of Life in Old Age*. Maidenhead: Open University Press.

Davie, G. (1994) *Religion in Britain Since 1945: Believing Without Belonging*. Oxford: Blackwell.

Davie, G. (1990) Believing without belonging: is this the future of religion in Britain? *Social Compass*, 37(4): 455–69.

Davie, G. and Vincent, J. (1998) Progress report religion and old age, *aging and Society*, 18: 101–10.

Dawes, T. and Thoner, G. (1998) aging and ethnicity, *Ethnicity and Health*, 3(4): 301–6.

Dean, M. (n.d.) *Growing Older in the 21st Century*, Swindon: ESRC.

Debate of the Age Health and Care Study Group (1999) *The Future of Health and Care of Older People: The Best is Yet to Come*. London: Age Concern.

De Beauvoir, S. (1970) *The Coming of Age*. London: Weidenfeld &

Nicholson.

De Jong Gierveld, J. (2003) Social networks and social well-being of older men and women living alone, in S. Arber, K. Davidson and J. Ginn (eds), *Gender and aging*. Maidenhead: Open University Press.

De Roover, J. (2004) Religious Tolerance: the History of a Christian Idea. Paper presented at the European Association for the Study of Religions Fourth Annual Conference, Santander, September.

Denzin, N. (1989) *Interpretive Interactionism,* in Applied Social Research Methods Series, 16. Thousand Oaks CA: Sage.

Department for Communities and Local Government (2006) *English House Condition Survey 2004: Annual Report*. London: Department for Communities and Local Government.

Department of Work and Pensions (DWP) (2005) *Women and Pensions: The Evidence*. Leeds: DWP.

Dhalech, M. (1999) *Challenging Racism in the Rural Idyll*. London: Citizens Advice Bureau.

Doyal, L., Harrison, L. and Charlwood, P. (eds) (1998) *Women and the National Health Service: A Case for Change?* Buckingham: Open University Press.

Dressel, P.L. and Barnhill, S.K. (1994) Reframing gerontological thought and practice: the case of grandmothers with daughters in prison, *The Gerontologist*, 34(5): 685–91.

Dunn, C. (1999) The effect of aging on autonomy, in A.H. Lesser (ed.), *aging, Autonomy and Resources*. Aldershot: Ashgate.

Durkheim, E. (1995) *The Elementary Forms of Religious Life*, trans. K.E. Fields. New York: Free Press.

Eldred, J. (2002) *Community, connection, and caring: towards a Christian feminist practical theology of older women*. Unpublished PhD thesis, University of Leeds.

Eley, G. and Suny, R.G. (eds) (1996) Introduction: from the moment of social history to the work of cultural representations, in G. Eley and R.G. Suny (eds), *Becoming National: A Reader*. New York: Oxford University Press.

Elias, N. (1985) *The Loneliness of the Dying*. Oxford: Basil Blackwell.

Elster, J. (1986*) Rational Choice*. Oxford: Blackwell.

Equal Opportunities Commission (2007) *Completing the Revolution*. Manchester: EOC.

Estes, C.L. (1979) *The Aging Enterprise*. San Francisco, CA: Jossey-Bass.

Estes, C.L., Gerard, L., Zones, J.S and Swan, J.S. (1984) *Political Economy, Health and aging*. Boston: Little Brown.

Estes, C.L. (2001) *Social Policy and Aging*. Thousand Oak: Sage.

Estes, C.L., Biggs, S. and Phillipson, C. (2003) *Social Theory, Social Policy and aging*. Maidenhead: Open University Press.

Evandrou, M. (2000) Social inequalities in later life: the socio-economic position of older people from ethnic minority groups in Britain, *Population Trends*, 101. London: TSO.

Evason, E. and Spence, L. (2002) *Women and Pensions*. Belfast: Equality Commission for Northern Ireland.

Featherstone, M. and Hepworth, M. (1991) The mask of aging and the postmodern lifecourse, in M. Featherstone, M. Hepworth and B.S. Turner (eds), *The Body, Social Process and Cultural Theory*. London: Sage.

Featherstone, M. and Hepworth, M. (1995) Images of positive aging: a case study of retirement choice magazine, in M. Featherstone and A. Wernick (eds), *Images of Aging*. London: Routledge.

Featherstone, M. and Hepworth, M. (2000) Images of aging, in J. Bond., P. Colemen and S. Peace (eds), *An Introduction to Social Gerontology*. London: Sage.

Field, D., Hockey, J. and Small, N. (eds) (1997) *Death, Gender and Ethnicity*. London: Routledge.

Finch, J. (1989) *Family Obligations and Social Change*. Cambridge: Polity.

Finch, J. (2000) Foreword, in M. Bernard, J. Phillips, L. Machin and V. Harding Davies (eds), *Women aging*. London: Routledge.

Finch, J. and Mason, J. (1993) *Negotiating Family Responsibilities*. London: Routledge.

Friedman, M. (1997) Autonomy and social relationships: rethinking the feminist critique, in D. Tietjens Meyers (ed.), *Feminists Rethink the Self*. Oxford: Westview Press.

Fine, M. et al. (eds) (1997) *Off White*. New York: Routledge.

Ford, J. and Sinclair, R. (1987) *Sixty Years On: Women Talk About Old Age*. London: Women's Press.

Foucault, M. (1979) *Discipline and Punish*. Harmondsworth: Penguin.

Frank, A.W. (1991) For a sociology of the body: an analytical review, in M. Featherstone, M. Hepworth and B.S. Turner (eds), *The Body, Social Process and Cultural Theory*. London: Sage.

Franks, M. (2000) Crossing the borders of whiteness? White Muslim women who wear the hijab in Britain today, *Journal of Ethnic and Racial Studies*, 23(5): 917–29.

Franks, M. (2001a) Shouting at God: some older Dominican women and empowerment. Paper presented at the DSA Women and Development Annual Conference, University of York, May.

Franks, M. (2001b) *Women and Revivalism in the West: Choosing 'Fundamentalisms' in a Liberal Democracy*. Houndmills: Palgrave.

Franks, M. (2002) Feminisms and cross-ideological feminist social research: standpoint, situatedness and positionality – developing cross-ideological feminist research, *Journal of International Women's Studies*, 3(2). Available at www.bridgew.edu/depts/artscnce/jiws/index.htm

Franks, M. (2004) *Before and after: the Hijab as a Focus of Religious Tolerance and Intolerance Prior to and Post 11th September 2001*. Paper presented at the EASR Fourth Annual Conference, Santander, September.

Franks, M. (2006) *Safeguarding and promoting the welfare of children in the African refugee community in Newcastle*. London: The Children's Society.

Franks, M. (in press) Islamic feminist strategies in a liberal democracy: how feminist are they? *Comparative Islamic Studies*. London: Equinox.

Franks, M. and Medforth, R. (2005) Young helpline callers and difference: exploring gender, ethnicity and sexuality in helpline access and provision, *Child and Family Social Work*, 10(1): 77–85.

Freedman, R. (1988) *Beauty Bound: Why Women Strive for Physical Perfection*. London: Columbus Books.

Furedi, F. (2004) *Therapy Culture: Cultivating Uncertainty in an Uncertain Age*. London: Routledge.

Gabriel, T. (2003) The United Nuwabian Nation of Moors, in C. Partridge (ed.), *UFO Religions*. London: Routledge.

Gannon, L.R. (1999) *Women and aging: Transcending the Myths*. London: Routledge.

Garvie, D. (2004) *The Black and Minority Ethnic Housing Crisis*. London: Shelter.

Gelfland, D.E. (1994) *aging and Ethnicity: Knowledge and Services*. New York: Springer Publishing Company.

Ghorashi, H. (2003) *Ways to Survive, Battles to Win: Iranian Women*

Exiles in the Netherlands and the United States. New York: Nova.

Gibson, P.A. (1999) African American grandmothers: new mothers again, *Affilia*, 14(3): 329–43.

Gilhooly, M., Hamilton, K., O'Neill, M. et al. (2003) Transport and aging: extending quality of life via public and private transport, *Growing Older Programme Research Finding*, 16. Sheffield: University of Sheffield.

Gilleard, C. and Higgs, P. (2000) *Cultures of aging.* Harlow: Pearson Educational Limited.

Gilliat-Ray, S. (2001) Sociological perspectives on the pastoral care of minority faiths in hospital, in H. Orchard (ed.), *Spirituality in Health Care Contexts*. London: Jessica Kingsley.

Ginn, J. (2003) *Gender, Pensions and the Lifecourse.* Bristol: Policy Press.

Ginn, J. and Arber, S. (1999) The politics of old age in the UK, in A. Walker and G. Naegele (eds), *The Politics of Old Age In Europe*. Buckingham: Open University Press.

Ginn, J. and Arber, S. (2000) Ethnic inequality in later life: variation in financial circumstances by gender and ethnic group, *Education and aging*, 15(1): 65–83.

Ginn, J. and Arber, S. (2001) A colder pension climate for British women, in J. Ginn, D. Street and S. Arber (eds), *Women, Work and Pensions*. Buckingham: Open University Press.

Ginn, J., Daly, M. and Street, D. (2001) Engendering pensions: a comparative framework, in J. Ginn, D. Street and S. Arber (eds), *Women, Work and Pensions*. Buckingham: Open University Press.

Ginn, J., Street, D. and Arber, S. (2001) *Women, Work and Pensions,* Buckingham: Open University Press.

Goffman, E. (1959) *The Presentation of Self in Everyday Life.* Garden City, NY: Doubleday.

Goffman, E. (1963) *Stigma: Notes on the Management of Spoiled Identity.* NJ: Spectrum/Prentice Hall.

Goffman, E. (1971) *Relations in Public: Microstudies of the Public Order.* London: Penguin.

Gorer, G.G. (1965) *Death, Grief and Mourning in Contemporary Britain.* London: Cresset.

Gouldner, A. (1960) The norm of reciprocity: a preliminary statement, *American Sociological Review*, 25: 161–78.

Graham, H. (2000) *Understanding Health Inequalities.* Buckingham:

Open University Press.

Grant, B.C. (2001) You're never too old: beliefs about physical activity and playing sport in later life, *aging and Society*, 21: 777–98.

Grimshaw, J. (1986) *Philosophy and Feminist Thinking*. London: University of Minnesota Press.

Gronvold, R.L. (1988) Measuring affectual solidarity, in D.J. Mangen, V.L. Bengtson and P.H. Landry Jr (eds), *Measurement of Intergenerational Relations*. Newbury Park, CA: Sage.

Grosz, E. (1994) *Volatile Bodies: Towards a Corporeal Feminism*. Indiana University Press.

Gurney, C. and Means, R. (1993) The meaning of home in later life, in S. Arber and M. Evandrou (eds), *aging, Independence and the Life Course*. London: Jessica Kingsley.

Hallberg, I.R. (2004) Death and dying from old people's point of view: A literature review, *Aging, Clinical and Experimental Research*, 16(2): 87–103.

Hanegraaff, W.J. (1999) New age spiritualities as secular religion: a historian's perspective, *Social Compass*, 46(2): 145–60.

Harding, S. (1991) *Whose Science? Whose Knowledge?*, Buckingham: Open University Press.

Hareven, T. (1982) Preface, in T. Hareven and K. Adams (eds), *aging and Life Course Transitions*. London: Tavistock.

Harper, S. (2000) aging update: aging 2000 – questions for the 21st century, *aging and Society*, 20: 111–22.

Harrison, J. (1983) Women and aging: experience and implications, *aging and Society*, 3(2): 209–35.

Hockey, J. and James, A. (1993) *Growing Up and Growing Old*. London: Sage.

Hazan, H. (1994) *Old Age: Constructions and Deconstructions*. Cambridge: Cambridge University Press.

Heikkinen, R.L. (2000) aging in an autobiographical context, *aging and Society*, 20: 467–83.

Heywood, F., Oldman, C. and Means, R. (2002) *Housing and Home in Later Life*. Buckingham: Open University Press.

Hill, D. and Tigges, L. (1995) Gendering welfare state theory: a cross-national study of women's public pension quality, *Gender and Society*, 9(1): 99–119.

Hockey, J. and James, A. (1993) *Growing Up and Growing Old: aging and Dependency in the Life Course*. London: Sage.

Hockey, J. and James, A. (2003) *Social Identities Across the Life Course*. London: Palgrave.

Holland, C. (ed.) (2005) *Recruitment and Sampling: Qualitative Research with Older People*. London: Centre for Policy on aging.

Holland, C., Kellaher, L., Peace, S. et al. (2005) Getting out and about, in A. Walker (ed.) *Understanding Quality of Life in Old Age*. Maidenhead: Open University Press.

Holstein, J. and Gubrium, J. (2000) *The Self We Live By*. Oxford: Oxford University Press.

Howarth, G. (2006) *Death and Dying: A Sociological Introduction*. Cambridge: Polity Press.

Hughes, B. (2000) Medicalized bodies, in Hancock, P. et al. *The Body, Culture and Society: An Introduction*. Buckingham: Open University Press.

Hurd, L. (1999) 'We're not old!' Older women's negotiation of aging and oldness, *Journal of aging Studies*, 13(4): 419–39.

Irwin, S. (1999) Later life, inequality and sociological theory, *aging and Society*, 19: 691–715.

Jamieson, A. and Victor, C.R. (eds) (2002) *Researching aging and Later Life*. Buckingham: Open University Press.

Jarvis, C., Hancock, R., Askham, J. and Tinker, A. (1996) *Getting Around at 60: A Profile of Britain's Older Population*. London: HMSO.

Jentsch, B. (1998) The interpreter 'effect': rendering interpreters visible in cross-cultural research and methodology, *Journal of European Social Policy*, 8(4): 275–89.

Jerrome, D. (1981) The significance of friendship for women in later life, *aging and Society*, 1(2): 175–97.

Jerrome, D. (1993a) *Good Company*, Edinburgh: Edinburgh University Press.

Jerrome, D. (1993b) Intimacy and sexuality among older women, in M. Bernard and K. Meade (eds), *Women Come of Age*. London: Edward Arnold.

Kabeer, N. (1999) Resources, agency, achievements: reflections on the measurement of women's empowerment, *Development and Change*, 30: 435–64.

Kalsi, S.S. (1992) *The Evolution of a Sikh Community in Britain: Reli-*

gious and Social Change Among the Sikhs of Leeds and Bradford, Community Religions Project Monographs. Leeds: University of Leeds, Department of Theology and Religious Studies

Karlsen, S. and Nazroo, J.Y. (2002) Agency and structure: the impact of ethnic identity and racism on the health of ethnic minority people, *Sociology of Health and Illness,* 24(1): 1–20.

Katbamna, S. (2004) *Perspectives on aging and Financial Planning for Old Age in South Asian Communities.* Leicester: University of Leicester.

Kaufman, S.R. (1986) *The Ageless Self: Sources of Meaning in Late Life.* Wisconsin: University of Wisconsin Press.

Keith, J., Fry, C.L. and Ikels, C. (1990) Community as context for successful aging, in Sokolovsky, J. (ed.), *The Cultural Context of aging.* London: Bergin and Garvey.

Khan, S. (1998) Muslim women: negotiations in the third space, *Signs: Journal of Women in Culture and Society,* 23(2): 464–94.

King, U. (1996) Spirituality, in Isherwood, L. and McEwan, D. (eds), *An A to Z of Feminist Theology.* Sheffield: Sheffield Academic Press.

Knott, K. (1998) Notions of destiny in women's self-construction, *Religion,* 28: 405–11.

Knott, K. (2005a) *The Location of Religion: A Spatial Analysis.* London: Equinox Publishing Ltd.

Knott, K. (2005b) Spatial theory and method for the study of religion, *Temenos: Nordic Journal of Comparative Religion,* 41(2): 153–84.

Knott, K. and Franks, M. (2007) Secular values and the location of religion: a spatial analysis of an English medical centre, *Health and Place,* 13(1). 224–37.

Koenig, H.G., Kuale, J.N. and Farrel, C. (1988) Religion and well-being in later life, *The Gerontologist,* 28: 18–28.

Kubler-Ross, E. (1970) *On Death and Dying.* London: Tavistock.

Kulchyski, P., McCaskill, D. and Newhouse, D. (1999) *In the Words of Elders: Aboriginal Cultures in Transition.* Toronto: University of Toronto Press.

Jocelyn-Armstrong, M. (2000) Older women's organization of friendship support networks: an African American-White American comparison, *Journal of Women and aging,* 12: 93–105.

Lader, D., Short, S. and Gershuny, J. (2006) *The Time Use Survey 2005: How We Spend Our Time.* London: ONS.

Laslett, P. (1987) The emergence of the third age, *Aging and Society,*

7(2): 133–60.

Laslett, P. (1989) *A Fresh Map of Life: The Emergence of the Third Age*. London: Weidenfeld & Nicholson.

Laslett, P. (1996) *A Fresh Map of Life: The Emergence of the Third Age*. 2nd edn. London: Macmillan.

Lawless, E.J. (1991) Women's life stories and reciprocal ethnography as feminist and emergent, *Journal of Folklore Research*, 28(1): 35–60.

Layder, D. (1998) *Sociological Practice*. London: Sage.

Lee, E. and Jackson, E. (2002) The pregnant body, in M. Evans and E. Lee (eds), *Real Bodies: A Sociological Introduction*. London: Palgrave.

Letherby, G. (2003) *Feminist Research in Theory and Practice*. Buckingham: Open University Press.

Levin, J.S. (ed.) (1994) *Religion and aging and health: theoretical foundations and methodological Frontiers*, Sage: London.

Lock, M. (1998) Anomalous aging: managing the postmenopausal body, *Body and Society*, 4(1): 35–61.

Lopata, H.Z. (1996) *Current Widowhood*. London: Sage.

Lovibond, S. (2001) 'Gendering' as an ethical concept, *Feminist Theory*, 2(2): 151–8.

Lowdell, C., Evandrou, M., Bardsley, M., Morgan, D. and Soljak, M. (2000) *Health of Ethnic Minority Elders in London*. London: Public Health Directorate.

Lowenthal, D. (1972) *West Indian Societies*. Oxford: Oxford University Press.

Lyon, W. (1995) Islam and Islamic women in Britain, *Woman: A Cultural Review*, 6(1): 46–56.

Mac an Ghaill, M. (1999) *Contemporary Racisms and Ethnicities*, Buckingham: Open University Press.

Mac an Ghaill, M. (2000) Debates: 'The Irish in Britain: the invisibility of ethnicity and anti-Irish racism', *Journal of Ethnic and Migration Studies*, 26(1): 137–47.

MacKinnon, C. (1989) *Towards a Feminist Theory of the State*. Cambridge, MA: Harvard University Press.

MacRobert, I. (1988) *The Black Roots and the White Racism of Early Pentecostalism in the USA*. Basingstoke: Macmillan.

Marcoen, A. (1994) Spirituality and personal well-being in old age, *aging and Society*, 14: 521–36.

Markides, K.S. (ed.) (1989) *aging and Health: Perspectives on Gender*,

Race, Ethnicity and Class, London: Sage.

Mauss, M. (1966) *The Gift: Forms and Functions of Exchange in Archaic Societies*. London: Cohen and West.

Maynard, M. (1999) What do older women want? in S. Walby (ed.), *New Agendas for Women*. London: Macmillan.

Maynard, M. (2002) Studying age, 'race' and gender: translating a research proposal into a project, *International Journal of Social Research Methodology*, 5(1): 31–40.

McClintock Fulkerson, M. (1996) Changing the subject, *Literature and Theology*, 10(2): 131–47.

McMunn, A., Breeze, E., Goodman, A., Nazroo, J. and Oldfield, Z. (2005) Social determinants of health in old age, in M. Marmot and R.G. Wilkinson (eds), *Social Determinants of Health*. Oxford: Oxford University Press.

Mellor, P.A. (1993) Reflexive traditions: Anthony Giddens, high modernity, and the contours of contemporary religiosity; *Religious Studies*, 29: 111–27.

Mellor, P.A. and Shilling, C. (1994) Reflexive modernity and the religious body, *Religion*, 24: 23–42.

Modood, T., Berthoud, R., Lakey, J. et al. (1997) *Ethnic Minorities in Britain: Diversity and Disadvantage*. London: Social Policy Studies Institute.

Moody, H.R. (1993) Overview: what is critical gerontology and why is it important?, in T.R. Cole, W.A. Achenbaum, P.L. Jacobi and P. Kastenbaum (eds), *Voices and Visions of Aging*. New York: Springer.

Morell, C.M. (2002) Empowerment and long-living women: a return to the rejected body, *Journal of Aging Studies*, 17(1):69–85.

Morgan, K. (ed.) (1992) *Gerontology: Responding to an aging Society*, London: Jessica Kingsley.

Morris, D.C. (1991) Church attendance, religious activities, and the life satisfaction of older adults in Middletown, USA, *Journal of Religious Gerontology*, 8(1).

Mouzelis, N. (1991) *Back to Sociological Theory*. London: Macmillan.

Nakayama, T. and Martin, J.N. (1999) (eds) *Whiteness: The Communication of Social Identity*. London: Sage.

National Statistics (2001) *The Classification of Ethnic Groups*, London: National Statistics.

National Statistics (2004) *Focus on Religion*, London: National Statistics.

Nazroo, J. (2004) Ethnic disparities in aging health: what can we learn from the United Kingdom?, in N. Anderson, R. Bulatao and B. Cohen (eds), *Critical Perspectives on Racial and Ethnic Differentials in Health in Later Life*. Washington, DC: National Academy Press.

Nazroo, J., Babekal, M., Blane, D. and Grewal, I. (2004) Ethnic inequalities, in A. Walker and C. Hagan Hennessy (eds), *Growing Older: Quality of Life in Old Age*. Maidenhead: Open University Press.

Nazroo, J., Bajekal, M., Blane, D. and Grewal, I. (2005) Ethnic inequalities in quality of life at older ages, in A. Walker with S. Northmore (eds), *Growing Older in a Black and Ethnic Minority Group*. London: Age Concern.

National Service Framework for Older People (2001). Available at http://www.gov.uk/PublicationsAndStatistics/Publications/Publications PolicyAndGuidance/PublicationsPolicyAndGuidanceArticle/fs/en? CONTENT_ ID4003066&chk=wg3bg0 (accessed 18 January 2006).

National Statistics (2006) *National Population Projections 2004-based*. London: National Statistics. Available at www.statistics.gov.uk/downloads/ theme_ population/PP2_No25.pdf

Niebor, A., Lindenberg, S., Boomsma, A. and Van Bruggen, A.C. (2005) Dimensions of well-being and their measurement: the SPF-Il scale, *Social Indicators Research*, 73: 313–53.

Oberg, P. (1996) The absent body – a social and gerontological paradox, *aging and Society, Special Issue: aging, Biography and Practice*, 16(6):701–19.

Office of the Deputy Prime Minister (ODPM) (2003) *Housing and Black and Minority (BME) Communities: Review of the Evidence Base*. London: ODPM.

ONS (2002) *Results from the 2001 Census Data*. London: Office for National Statistics.

ONS (2003) *Census 2001*. London: TSO.

ONS (2004) *Social Trends 34*. London: The Stationery Office.

ONS (2005) *Office of National Statistics Mid-2004 Population Estimates*. Available at: www.statistics.gov.uk/statbase/explorer.asp?CTG=3&SL =4819&D= 4912&DCT=32&DT=32#4912

Ousley, H. (2001) *Community Pride Not Prejudice*. Bradford: Bradford Vision.

Owen, D. (1996) Size, structure and growth of the ethnic minority populations, in D. Coleman and J. Salt (eds), *Ethnicity in the Census, 1*. London: HMSO.

Patel, N. (1999) *aging Matters, Ethnic Concerns*. London: Age Concern.

Pattillo-McCoy, M. (1998) Church culture as a strategy of action in the black community, *American Sociological Review*, 63(6): 767–84.

Peat, M. (2004) Second fiddle or second chance? The significance of grandfatherhood. Unpublished PhD thesis, University of York.

Peniston Bird, C. and Summerfield, P. (2007) *Contesting Home Defence: Men, Women and the Home Guard in the Second World War*. Manchester: Manchester University Press.

Penn, R., Favell, A. and Cross, M. (2000) *Review Symposium of Ethnic Minorities in British Social Science: Three Views*, 26(2): 357–67.

Pensions Policy Institute (2003) *The Under-pensioned Ethnic Minorities*. London: PPI.

Peterson, A. and Bunton, R. (1997) *Foucault, Health and Medicine*. London: Routledge.

Phillipson, C. (1982) *Capitalism and the Construction of Old Age*. London: Macmillan.

Phillipson, C. (1998) *Reconstructing Old Age*. London: Sage.

Phillipson, C., Bernard, M., Phillips, J. and Ogg, J. (2001) *The Family and Community Life of Older People*. London: Routledge.

Phillipson, C. (2004) Globalisation. Paper presented at the 17th IAG Conference, Vancouver. Available at: www.keele.ac.uk/depts/so/csg/globalisation.htm (accessed 20 July 2004).

Platteau, J.-P. (2000) *Institutions, Social Norms and Economic Development*. Newark, NJ: Harwood Academic Publishers.

Platteau, J.-P. (2004) Order, the rule of law and moral norms, in J. Toye (ed.), *Trade and Development: Directions for the Twenty-first Century*. Cheltenham: Edward Elgar.

Plaza, D. (2000) Transnational grannies: the changing family responsibilities of elderly African-Caribbean-born women resident in Britain, *Social Indicators Research*, 51: 75105.

Posner, R.A. (1995) *aging and Old Age*. London: University of Chicago Press.

Pulsipher, L.M. (1992) Changing roles in the life cycles of women in traditional West Indian houseyards, in J.H. Momsen (ed.), *Women and Change: A Pan-Caribbean Perspective*. London: James Currey.

Pulsipher, L.M. (1993) He won't let she stretch she foot': gender relations in traditional West Indian houseyards, in C. Katz and J. Monk (eds), *Full Circles*. London: Routledge.

Qureshi, H. and Walker, A. (1989) *The Caring Relationship: Elderly People and their Families*. Basingstoke: Macmillan.

Ram-Prasad, C. (1995) A classical Indian philosophical perspective on aging and the meaning of life, *aging and Society*, 15: 1–36.

Reynolds, T. (2002) On relations between black female researchers and participants, in T. May (ed.), *Qualitative Research in Action*. London: Sage.

Robertson, A. (1999) Beyond apocalyptic dependency: towards a moral economy of interdependence, in M. Minkler and C.L. Estes (eds), *Critical Gerontology: Perspectives from Political and Moral Economy*. Amityville, NY: Baywood Publishing Co.

Robertson Elliot, F. (1996) *Gender, Family and Society*. Basingstoke: Macmillan.

Rose, N. (1999). Cambridge: *Powers of Freedom: Reframing Political Thought*, Cambridge: Cambridge University Press.

Rouse, R. (1995) Questions of identity: personhood and collectivity in transnational migration to the United States, *Critique of Anthropology*, 15(4): 351–80.

Rowlands, J. (1997) What is empowerment? in H. Afshar and F. Alikhan (eds), *Empowering Women for Development*. Hyderabad, India: Booklinks Corporation.

Rowlands, J. (1998) A word of the times, in H. Afshar (ed.), *Women and Empowerment*. London: Macmillan.

Sapp, S. (1987) An alternative Christian view of aging, *Journal of Religion and Aging*, 4:1.

Scharf, T. (2005) Recruiting older research participants: lessons from deprived neighbourhoods, in C. Holland (ed.), *Recruitment and Sampling: Qualitative Research with Older People*. London: Centre for Policy on aging.

Scharf, T., Phillipson, C. and Smith, A.E. (2005) Social exclusion of older people in deprived urban communities of England, *European Journal of aging*, 2(2): 76–87.

Schmidt, G. (2002) Dialectics of authenticity: examples of ethnification of Islam amongst young Muslims in Sweden and the United States, *The Muslim World*, 92(1/2): 1–17.

Scott, J.C. (1976) *The Moral Economy of the Peasant: Rebellion and*

Subsistence in Southeast Asia. New Haven, Con: Yale University Press.

Scott, A. and Wenger, C. (1995) Gender and social support networks in later life, in S. Arber and J. Ginn (eds), *Connecting Gender and aging.* Buckingham: Open University Press.

Seale, C. (1998) *Constructing Death: The Sociology of Dying and Bereavement.* Cambridge: Cambridge University Press.

Siddell, M. (1993) Health issues and the older woman, in M. Bernard and K. Meade (eds), *Women Come of Age.* London: Edward Arnold.

Siddell, M. (1994) Death, dying and bereavement, in J. Bond, P. Coleman and S. Peace (eds), *aging in Society* London: Sage.

Siddell, M. (1995) *Health in Old Age.* Buckingham: Open University Press.

Sin, C.H. (2003) Interviewing in 'place': the socio-spatial construction of interview data, *Area,* 35(3): 305–12.

Sin, C.H. (2005) Sampling minority ethnic older people in Britain, *aging and Society,* 24: 257–77.

Singh, R. (2000) *Sikhs and Sikhism in Britain: Fifty Years on the Bradford Perspective.* Bradford: Bradford Libraries.

Skucha, J. and Bernard, M. (2000) 'Women's work' and the transition to retirement, in M. Bernard, J. Phillips, L. Machin and V. Harding Davies (eds), *Women aging,* London: Routledge.

Skucha, J. and Bernard, M. (eds) (2002) *Women aging.* London: Routledge.

Smith, A.E. (2000a) Quality of life: a review, *Education and aging,* 15 (3): 419–35.

Smith, A. (2000b) *Researching quality of life of older people: concepts, measures and findings,* working paper no. 7, Centre for Social Gerontology.

Smith, A.E. (2001) Defining quality of life, *ESRC's Growing Older Programme Newsletter,* Issue 2.

Sointu, E. (2005) The rise of an ideal: tracing changing discourses of well being, *The Sociological Review,* 53: 255–74.

Somerville, P. and Steele, A. (eds) (2001) *'Race', Housing and Social Exclusion.* London: Jessica Kingsley.

Sontag, S. (1978) The double standard of aging, in V. Carver and P. Liddiard (eds), *An aging Population.* Milton Keynes: Open University Press.

Stack, C.B. (1974) *All Our Kin: Strategies for Survival in a Black*

Community. New York: Harper Row.

Street, D. and Ginn, J. (2001) The demographic debate: the gendered political economy of pensions, in J. Ginn, D. Street and S. Arber (eds), *Women, Work and Pensions*. Buckingham: Open University Press.

Summerfield, P. (1989) *Women Workers in the Second World War: Production and Patriarchy in Conflict*. London: Routledge.

Summerfield, P. (1998) *Reconstructing Women's Wartime Lives: Discourse and Subjectivity in Oral Histories of the Second World War*. Manchester: Manchester University Press.

Sutcliffe, S.J. (2003) *Children of the New Age*, London: Routledge.

Tapper, N. (1991) *Bartered Brides: Politics, Gender and Marriage in Afghan Tribal Society*. Cambridge: Cambridge University Press.

Temple, B. (1997) Watch your tongue: issues in translation and cross-cultural research, *Sociology*, 31(3), 607–18.

Temple, B. and Edwards, R. (2002) Interpreters/translators and cross-cultural research: reflexivity and border crossings, *International Journal of Qualitative Methods*, 1, 2. Article 1. Available at: www.ualberta.ca/~ijqm/ (accessed 2 September 2007).

Thane, P. (2002) *Old Age in English History*. Oxford: Oxford University Press.

The Times (2005) *The Times Online*, 9 August.

The World Health Organization (1998) *Health for All Policy Framework for the European Region for the 21st Century*. Available at: www.euro.who.int/Governance/resolutions/1998/20030430_9, (accessed June 2006).

The World Health Organization (2002) *Active aging: A Policy Framework*. Available at: www.euro.who.int/document/hea/eactage polframe.pdf (accessed: 18 January 2006).

Thompson, P., Itzin, C. and Abendstern, M. (1990) *I Don't Feel Old*. Oxford: Oxford University Press.

Thuen, F. et al. (1997) The effect of widowhood on psychological wellbeing and social support in the oldest groups of the elderly, *Journal of Men's Health*, 6: 265–74.

Torres, S. (1999) A culturally-relevant theoretical framework for the study of successful aging, *aging and Society*, 19(1): 33–51.

Torres, S. (2003) A preliminary empirical test of the culturally-relevant theoretical framework for the study of successful aging, *Journal of*

Cross-cultural Gerontology, 18: 73–91.

Toulis, N.R. (1997) *Believing Identity: Pentecostalism and the Mediation of Jamaican Identity and Gender in England*. Oxford: Berg.

Townsend, P. (1981) The structured dependency of the elderly: a creation of social policy in the twentieth century, *aging and Society*, 1(1): 5–28.

Twyman, C., Morrison, J. and Sporton, D. (1999) The final fifth: autobiography, reflexivity and interpretation in cross-cultural research, *Area*, 31(4), 313–25.

Vermeulen, H. and Govers, C. (1994) Introduction, in H. Vermeulen and C. Govers (eds), *The Anthropology of Ethnicity: Beyond Ethnic Groups and Boundaries*, Amsterdam: Het Spinhuis.

Vincent, J. (2003) *Old Age*. London: Routledge.

Vom Bruck, G. (1997) Elusive bodies: the politics of aesthetics among Yemeni elite women, *Signs: Journal of Women in Culture and Society*, 23(1).

Walker, A. (1981) Towards a political economy of old age, *aging and Society*, 1 (1), 73–94.

Walker, A. (ed.) (1996) *The New Generational Contract*. London: UCL Press.

Walker, A. (2001) Presentation at the Launch Conference of the ESRC Growing Older Programme, March.

Walter, T. (1994) *The Revival of Death*. London: Routledge.

Walter, T. (1996) *The Eclipse of Eternity: A Sociology of the Afterlife*. Basingstoke: Macmillan.

Walter, T. (1999) *On Bereavement: The Culture of Grief*. Buckingham: Open University Press.

Webster, W. (1998) *Imagining Home: Gender, 'Race' and National Identity 1945–64*. London: UCL Press.

White, A. (2002) *Social Focus on Ethnic Minorities*. London: Office for National Statistics.

Williams, B. and Barlow, J.H. (1998) Falling out with my shadow: arthritis, in S. Nettleton, and J. Watson (eds), *The Body in Everyday Life*. London: Routledge.

Wilson, G. (2000) *Understanding Old Age*. London: Sage.

Woodward, K. (2003) You and me, us and them: issues of identity, in K. Woodward (ed.), *Social Sciences: The Big Issues*. London: Routledge.

Wouters, C. (2002) The quest for new rituals in dying and mourning:

changes in the we-I balance, *Body and Society*, 8(1): 1–27.

Wray, S. (2003) Women growing older: agency, ethnicity and culture, *Sociology*, 37(3): 511–28.

Wray, S. (2004) What constitutes agency and empowerment for women in later life? *The Sociological Review*, 52(1): 22–38.

Wray, S. and Bartholomew, M. (2006) Older African-Caribbean women: the influence of migration on experiences of health and well-being in later life, *Journal of Research, Policy and Planning*, 18(2):104–20.

Wray, S. (2007) Health, exercise and well-being: the experiences of midlife women from diverse ethnic backgrounds, *Social Theory and Health*, 5(2): 126–44.

Wright, A. (2000) *Spirituality and Education*. London and New York: Routledge/Falmer.

Index